SHIATSU
FOR BEGINNERS
A STEP-BY-STEP GUIDE

NIGEL DAWES

PIATKUS

To my parents for their love and support
over the years

Note to the reader

This book is a beginners' guide to the practice of some basic Shiatsu techniques. It is not intended as a thorough explanation of the theory and practice of Shiatsu as a therapy. Whilst every effort has been made to illustrate each technique clearly and carefully, there can be no substitute for the supervision of a qualified teacher of Shiatsu. The author and the publisher disclaim all responsibility for any accident or injury caused by any inappropriate use of the techniques shown in this book.

Copyright © 1991 Nigel Dawes

First published in 1991 by
Judy Piatkus (Publishers) Ltd of
5 Windmill Street, London W1P 1HF

Originally published as
The Shiatsu Workbook

Reprinted 1994

*The moral right of the author
has been asserted*

A catalogue record for this book is available
from the British Library

ISBN 0–7499–1073–9 hbk
ISBN 0–7499–1068–2 pbk

Edited by Esther Jagger
Designed by Paul Saunders
Photography by Yona Zaloscer

Typeset in Lasercomp Sabon
Printed and bound in Great Britain by
Butler & Tanner Ltd, Frome and London

CONTENTS

Acknowledgements

I would like to thank the following for their contribution in making this book possible.

Firstly, all those who influenced my training in oriental medicine including Todo sensei, Nagura sensei, Hirai sensei, Dr Yom, Dr Gao, Peter Townsend, Marcus Bachino, Gretchen De Soriano and especially my Shiatsu teachers, Edward Bailey, Kaoru Kasugai, Kimura sensei, Endo sensei and most of all, Suzuki sensei.

All the various people who made the photos come alive, notably Camden Studios, Stirling Cooper for the wardrobe, Tinks Reding and Georgie Eyre for the excellent make-up, Penny Southgate, Julia Dell and Atif Dar for being great models, Roy Reed for his expert technical advice and especially Yona Zaloscer for her sensitive and inspired photography.

All the many people who helped inspire me to produce this book from Margaret Adolphus who encouraged me to write it in the first place through to the wonderful team at Piatkus Books who agreed to publish it, especially Anne Lawrance who quietly supported me throughout, Esther Jagger who did the final editing, Paul Saunders for his brilliant artistic design and Gill Cormode who was an ever-patient and inspiring editor.

Finally, to all my friends and family who have had to put up with me while this book has been in the making, especially my wife, Felicity, without whose support and encouragement I would never have completed it!

ABOUT THE AUTHOR

Nigel Dawes is a UK citizen, educated in France and England, now living in the USA. He graduated from Cambridge University with an MA in Modern Languages and Literature before travelling to Japan and China, spending five years studying Oriental Medicine and philosophy.

Having graduated from schools in Tokyo and Peking, he returned to Britain in 1987 to begin a practice combining Shiatsu, Acupuncture and Chinese Herbs. At the same time, he founded The London College of Shiatsu of which he is Principal.

His clinical and teaching work has taken him all over Britain, to the Middle East where he teaches regularly in Israel and, most recently, to New York.

His interests include travel, Tai Chi Chuan, Zen Meditation and writing. This is his second book.

FOREWORD

In the Western world our approach to healthcare is too often based on the 'quick fix' solution. The focus is on *disease control* rather than *health maintenance* and responsibility is taken out of the hands of the individual and surrendered to the professional. Shiatsu is one way in which we can reclaim responsibility for ourselves.

For centuries, Asian medicine has stressed the importance of preventative medicine, in the belief that good health is synonymous with balance in all aspects of our lives. Health practices, such as Shiatsu, are therefore aimed at achieving this balance in our bodies. Shiatsu is a form of oriental massage along the body's energy channels or meridians which balances the body's energies and leads to an increased sense of wellbeing and vitality.

In *Shiatsu for Beginners* I aim to convey a sense of the art of Shiatsu in language and pictures. I want to teach you the basic techniques so that you can use your newly-learned skills on your friends and family to mutual benefit. Shiatsu will promote freedom and equanimity of movement, concentration and focus, balance and coordination. It can also be used to strengthen the body's resistance to illness and help many everyday ailments such as headaches, backaches, sciatica, fatigue, cramps, poor circulation and so on.

If you have already received and enjoyed a Shiatsu treatment and are curious to find out more about the background and principles of practice, this book will be invaluable. But the real value of this book lies in opening you up to a whole new aspect of communication through touch which has the power to create balance and peace in our busy lives. This is a true gift to give or receive.

Nigel Dawes
January 1994

What is Shiatsu?

DEFINITION

'Shiatsu' is a Japanese word made up of two written characters meaning 'finger' (*shi*) and 'pressure' (*atsu*). It is used to describe a form of manipulative therapy, recognised by the Japanese government, which focuses on the use of static pressure applied to specific points and lines all over the body. These points, called *'tsubo'* in Japanese, are also used in acupuncture and are sometimes called 'acupoints' in English. The lines along which most of the points are located are known as 'meridians'; also common to the theory and practice of other oriental disciplines such as acupuncture and herbal medicine.

Not surprisingly then, Shiatsu is often called 'acupressure', and stimulation of the points with pressure is certainly one of the techniques used – though not the only nor even the principal one. In fact, pressure is applied to wide areas as well as precise points all over the body, using not only the fingers and thumbs but also the palms, elbows, knees and feet. In addition to the pressure itself, gentle stretch and manipulation techniques are used which probably owe more to modern physiotherapy than to traditional oriental massage. At times, very light 'holding' techniques may be used, usually with the palm – almost like the laying on of hands in spiritual healing.

So in practice, modern Shiatsu incorporates a mixture of different approaches, mostly involving pressure; some are based on ancient methods, others on more recent ones, but all share a common element – touch. Shiatsu, then, is first and foremost a 'hands-on' therapy.

ORIGINS AND HISTORY

Clearly, the origins of Shiatsu lie in the natural response to injury, pain or discomfort – to rub the affected area feels comforting and often relieves the pain. From this automatic response to dis-ease in the body there probably evolved, through trial and error, a systematic approach to the relief of certain ailments by concentrating on certain key areas and points which were observed to trigger specific repeatable results. Originally this was likely to have been done in an intuitive manner; but, over time, theories developed which tried to explain such phenomena. These theories (discussed in the next chapter) became the basis of a healthcare system which has remained in practical use for several thousand years in the East, and to which Shiatsu belongs.

In the earliest recorded Chinese medical text, *The Yellow Emperor's Classic of Internal Medicine*, written over two thousand years ago, the origins and development of different medical disciplines was attributed to the different regions of China: geography, diet and lifestyle varied enormously between these regions, and so did disease patterns. Thus acupuncture, massage and herbal medicine evolved side by side to treat the range of diseases encountered. The traditional massage of ancient China was known as 'Anmo' and found its way to Japan to be adopted and adapted by the Japanese, who called it 'Anma'.

In Japan, 'Anma' became a profession often associated with blind people and enjoyed an excellent reputation for several hundred years; however, as Western medical influences began to make their mark in the nineteenth century, it began to be looked down upon as folklore. Not until this century did people start to re-evaluate their traditional medical systems, and only after the Second World War in Japan and the appearance of Chairman Mao in China did these systems begin to re-establish themselves seriously.

SHIATSU TODAY

The term 'Shiatsu' is relatively new and represents only part of the original 'Do In Ankyo' system, which involved a comprehensive range of exercise, diet, meditation, massage, manipulation and pressure. The recent introduction of elements of physiotherapy reflects the influence of some Western approaches in modern Japan where Shiatsu is gradually regaining stature, though frankly is still viewed as old-fashioned by most Japanese today.

It is in Western countries that Shiatsu is really coming into its own as a respected therapy and, despite the initial fashionable prestige of being yet another 'mysterious oriental practice', it has taken a more widespread hold among the general public and is being enjoyed by thousands in Europe and North America for the prevention and treatment of many common ailments. It is enjoying a particular upsurge in popularity in Britain. Shiatsu is mostly available as private treatment in multi-disciplinary complementary health clinics or at home, but there are many examples of Shiatsu being used in hospital settings on the National Health and of GPs referring patients directly to practitioners. The role of Shiatsu within the healthcare system, public and private, is therefore in the process of developing rapidly in response to a genuine demand for this type of safe, effective therapy.

The Principles of Shiatsu

THE ROLE OF SHIATSU

I have already mentioned in the first chapter that the term 'Shiatsu' includes a number of different manipulative techniques from varying traditions. But the basic principles which govern its practice come from the classics of oriental medicine and form part of an integrated system of healthcare that has been in use for centuries. Just as in acupuncture or herbal medicine, Shiatsu employs its own system of diagnosis and treatment based on those principles. An outline of the way that Shiatsu works is useful for anyone learning to give it, in terms of both their understanding and their ability to share it with others. What follows is a simplified overview of a rich tapestry of knowledge based on several thousand years of empirical observation in the arts and sciences, and acquiring this depth of knowledge could become a lifetime preoccupation.

ORIENTAL MEDICINE AND THE ORIENTAL MIND

As Westerners looking at how oriental societies have traditionally viewed health and sickness, we need to take into account a basic paradox. In trying to get to grips with their medical theories we will naturally use a quite rational, logical approach which is unlikely to reveal anything to us: the more we try to understand how oriental medicine works, the less will be revealed. This is not to say that Eastern thinking is illogical – it simply follows different rules from our own. In his three-volume series *The Chinese Mind, The Indian Mind* and *The Japanese Mind*, Charles A. Moore points to the relationship between the individual and the universal as symbolising this basic difference. In both language and logic, people from the Eastern Hemisphere tend to express themselves in terms of universal concepts rather than individual ideas. The characters of their written languages suggest general ideas through pictures, whilst in their speech and body language they rely on intuition and suggestion rather than direct expression. Things are rarely thought of or expressed in black and white terms – there is no exact word for 'Yes' or 'No' in Japanese, for example.

It is not surprising, then, that modern scientific medicine, which does not recognise anything that cannot be clearly explained by logical means, is suspicious of the traditional systems of the East. Superstition and folklore were, after all, despised by the new logic which emerged from post-Renaissance Europe, and much of our own traditional knowledge of medicine was lost at that time. Oriental societies, however, have retained much of their traditional approach to health intact.

Eastern medicine developed directly from philosophy, which itself was based on an understanding of the nature of the universe. After observing certain natural laws in action it was thought that they could be used to understand the nature of living things, including human beings and the way they functioned. The theories that evolved from this empirical process were an attempt to express the particular through the general, but at all levels material phenomena were seen as interconnected and indivisible. As a result, such theories often appear vague and illogical to the Western mind.

Mind, Body and Spirit

The first and most basic feature of the oriental approach to health and disease is to consider the mind and body as an inseparable unit. Included in this is the dimension we could call 'spirit', which, regardless of religious faith, is believed to link the physical part of us with something metaphysical and universal. The Eastern concept of interconnectedness means that to the oriental mind a thought or feeling might produce a physical change, or vice versa. Anything from the movement of the planets to changes of season, climate, diet and lifestyle is considered to affect the individual to an equal degree.

This 'holistic' perception of the individual naturally encouraged philosophers and, later, physicians to express health as a function of the proper balance of all these different dimensions of human being. Early health practices therefore concentrated on disciplines which spanned all these dimensions – physical exercise, diet, fasting and meditation on a day-to-day basis, and other practices such as divination and astrology to guide the individual as to their wider purpose. The main focus of oriental medicine is therefore preventative in nature.

But if the individual was seen to be so inextricably linked with his or her internal and external environment, how could specific phenomena like a particular illness be interpreted? In disease as in health, the oriental mind takes the overview first and sees illness in very general terms. *The Yellow Emperor's Classic of Internal Medicine* asserts that 'those who rebel against the rules of the universe sever their own roots and ruin their true selves ...'. In order to describe these rules, a simple, dualistic model was used which allowed definition by comparison.

Yin and Yang

The principles used in the model were termed 'Yin', meaning dark or shade, and 'Yang', meaning bright or light. Just as the sun is bright, so it casts a shadow of darkness to which it is linked in a complementary but opposite way. These two polarities are used to describe all phenomena in nature, by ascribing different qualities to each. For example, Yang qualities are generally associated with more active, outward, strong, visible phenomena than Yin qualities, which usually describe more quiet, hidden, inward and powerful (in the sense of nourishing) phenomena. The relationship of Yin and Yang is governed by certain specific laws which had been observed at work in nature:

1. They are an expression of the infinite whole, the universe (e.g. each cell forms part of the whole body).

2. Their interaction produces all things (e.g. male and female produce new life).

3. They oppose each other but cannot exist without each other (e.g. the palm of your hand and the back of your hand).

4. They give to and support each other, but also take from and consume each other (e.g. parent and child relationship).

5. In extremes they can transform into their opposite (e.g. the changing seasons).

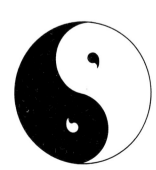

In medicine they are used to categorise the location, depth and nature of disease. More specifically, each sympton in turn can be compared in terms of Yin and Yang; this helps with both the diagnosis and prognosis of a disease. For example, a Yang disease is said to be acute and active, with symptoms likely to show up on the surface of the body and which are easily seen. Such symptoms are characterised by their strong nature, such as aches and pains, fever, dry throat and strong cough. A Yin disease, by contrast, has symptoms which are often hidden inside the body and are difficult to see. They may be only slight, but often persist and may be difficult to treat. In practice, as with the sun and its shadow, Yin and Yang diseases are closely linked and each may contain elements of the other. These polarities, as well as their relativity, are clearly suggested by the well-known symbol for Yin and Yang, showing a balance of equal and opposite forces each with an element of the other contained within it.

As in pathology, so in anatomy and physiology, Yin and Yang are used to describe the structure and function of the body. For example, the skin would be seen as more Yang (surface) than the internal organs, which would be more Yin (deep). However, this is not the same as saying that the skin *is* Yang, since it would in turn be more Yin than, say, the body hair. So the description is always relative.

Organ function, too, is described in terms of Yin and Yang. The so-called 'hollow' organs – the stomach, intestines and bladders – are considered more Yang (active and strong) compared to the 'solid' or vital organs – the heart, liver, kidney, spleen and lungs, which are more Yin in function (static, powerful and nourishing). The complementary aspect of Yin and Yang is symbolised by the special functional relationship enjoyed by specific pairs of organs, for example the kidney and bladder; the liver and gall bladder; the spleen and stomach; the lungs and large intestine; and the heart and small intestine.

Similarly, and more importantly in oriental medicine, the strength and constitution of the individual can be described in terms of Yin and Yang. This is done by describing the relative state of energy as being either 'Jitsu', meaning 'full' in Japanese, or 'Kyo', meaning 'empty'. Jitsu is a more Yang phenomenon, and Kyo is more Yin. Jitsu indicates strength in terms of physical condition, while Kyo suggests weakness. This is important as most oriental medicine, including Shiatsu, aims at mobilising the individual's own ability to recover from illness by themselves. Naturally a strong person, with more energy to spare, is likely to respond better to this kind of approach than a weak one. A truly depleted person is difficult to treat with Shiatsu alone; other methods, especially herbal medicine, in which something substantial is added to the body, may be required.

The Five Transformations

Just as the spinning ball of energy (the universe) was cleft into the polarities of Yin and Yang, so, gradually, certain elements in nature began gathering in certain distinct forms such as earth, metal, water, wood and fire. These elements were characterised, like Yin and Yang, by constant movement and change and were inter-related in similar ways. Some were observed to give rise to others, whilst equally they could do damage to another. For example, water naturally nourishes growth, symbolised by wood, though it can equally well extinguish fire. (The nature of these relationships is shown in the diagram at the top of page 12.)

In medicine, the basic energetic nature of each element, for

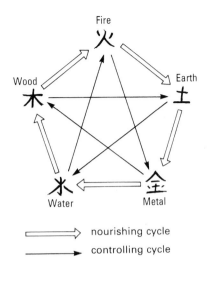

Fire 火

Wood 木

Earth 土

Water 水

Metal 金

⟹ nourishing cycle
⟶ controlling cycle

Five Elements	Human Body				
	Yin Organ	Yang Organ	Five Sense Organs	Five Tissues	Emotions
Wood	Liver	Gall Bladder	Eye	Tendon	Anger
Fire	Heart	Small Intestine	Tongue	Vessel	Joy
Earth	Spleen	Stomach	Mouth	Muscle	Meditation
Metal	Lung	Large Intestine	Nose	Skin and hair	Grief and melancholy
Water	Kidney	Urinary Bladder	Ear	Bone	Fright and fear

Five Transformations Table of Correspondences

example the nourishing energy of earth, was linked with the function of each of the Yin–Yang pairs of organs mentioned previously. In the example, the earth element would include spleen (which covers the pancreas function) and stomach – both organs of digestion, which thus provide the basic nourishing energy for the body.

Similar correspondences were established for other parts and functions of the body, describing anatomy and physiology as Yin and Yang do and thus providing a model to assess the causes and effects as well as the treatment of disease. Some of these correspondences are shown above. For example, when the fire energy is well balanced in the body the complexion is rosy, the vessels strong and the pumping action good, and the person will be joyful and happy. When this element is out of balance, the face may be flushed, the vessels clogged, the blood pressure affected and the person may be sad and depressed. Although this is very general description of some of the effects of heart disease, the associations are clear – and we know, for example, that heart attacks occur more often in the heat of the summer.

The model of the five transformations can be added to that of Yin and Yang in providing a basis for understanding how the oriental peoples saw the inter-relationships between the body functions both in health and in sickness. This of course is helpful in explaining disease, but more significantly in predicting it, which is what most oriental methods aim at doing. *The Yellow Emperor's Classic of Internal Medicine* says that 'the superior physician helps before the early budding of the disease ...'.

Most usefully, the five-transformation model highlights clear distinctions between energy types, which we can use to characterise personalities, constitutions and illnesses. But what exactly do the orientals mean by energy, and how is it transmitted in the body?

'Ki' Energy

The word 'Ki' in Japanese ('Chi' in Chinese) has a variety of meanings. Its most common translation is 'energy', as seen in words like 'Tenki', literally meaning 'heaven energy' and referring to the weather, or in the phrase 'O genki desu ka?' meaning literally 'And how is your Ki today?' – in other words, 'How are you?' But it also simply means 'air' or 'gas' and can refer to the air we breathe and the breath itself.

In any event, the concept of Ki suggests something vital which characterises movement and change, like energy itself, of which the two most obvious manifestations are Yin and Yang. As we have seen, they are in a state of perpetual motion and transformation; and life, including human life, occurs as a result of their interaction. Similarly, the five elements which make up the material world, as we have seen, are clear examples of 'Ki' manifesting in different forms.

Inside the body, energy manifests in Yin and Yang forms and in each of the five elemental phases as a constant state of exchange and transformation. This can vary from substantial, nourishing forms of energy like the blood, body fluids and tissues which are more Yin compared to more rarified, functional forms like gases and the 'Ki' that circulates in the meridians. In turn, such gases are absorbed into the bloodstream, transform and become relatively more Yin, only to return to a more Yang state as they are burnt up as fuel by the muscles.

Similarly, within the organ and meridian systems energy is constantly being exchanged according to the laws of the support and control cycles of the five transformations, so that the energy circulates to fill areas where it is lacking (Kyo) and drain off areas where it is excessive (Jitsu). The entire system is therefore designed to be self-regulating, which is why most imbalances correct themselves without effort. Treatment is only required for stubborn and persistent blockage or lack of energy in a certain area, which is where Shiatsu and related disciplines come in.

In fact, as I have mentioned, treatment for imbalances in the energy system which had already manifested as disease was considered inferior medicine; the superior physician would have treated such imbalance before it had a chance to appear. The simplest forms of such preventative treatment involved the proper use and combination of the most obvious Yin and Yang forms of energy freely available to human beings – food and air (oxygen). Hence the very earliest forms of preventative healthcare focused on diet and fasting (learning to control the nourishing Yin energies of the body) and on exercise and breathing (learning to manipulate the functional Yang energies of the body).

The Meridians

The method by which the orientals believed all energy circulated and nourished the whole person was through specific pathways, or meridians as they are usually called. The written characters meaning 'meridian' suggest the idea of a criss-cross network of interconnected pathways which link the organs, skin, flesh, muscle and bones in a unified body. The Ki that circulates within them may be more Yang in nature, defending the body on the outside, or more Yin in nature, nourishing the body on the inside. In any event, these channels run from deep in the organs out through major meridian branches to smaller and smaller ones, ending up at the outside of the body in the skin; then they go back again, just like the pattern of other major body systems such as the nervous and blood systems.

Each of the meridians was classified as Yin and Yang in nature depending on whether it connected with a Yin or Yang organ, and so it became known by the name of its associated organ. For example the liver meridian, which includes the liver organ, is Yin in nature and pertains to the wood element (see the table on page 12 for these correspondences). The flow of energy throughout the meridian system as a whole follows a specific sequence (see page 15) and is usually seen as beginning with the lungs, where energy is first taken into the body through the breath.

Because the meridians serve the whole body from outside in and inside out, they have a protecting role in stopping harmful energies from entering (in the form of bacteria and viruses); and they can also reflect the presence of harmful energy already inside the body in the form of symptoms on the outside. These may be felt as aches, pains, heat or cold, and in Shiatsu may be located as areas of

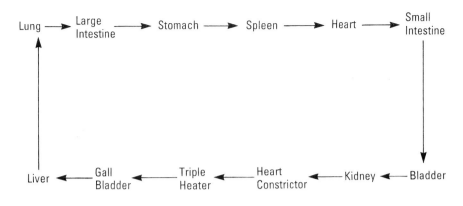

Energy Flow through the Meridians

particular sensitivity or tenderness. Finding these areas is one of the aims of Shiatsu diagnosis and treatment, since their quality and location can tell us a great deal about the origin, location and depth of an imbalance in the entire energy system, which will result in a given disease. The unique nature of the meridians is to reflect this kind of imbalance and then to act as the channel by which the imbalance can be corrected. In the case of Shiatsu, the affected meridian or points are worked on directly until proper energy flow is restored. This is the origin of a commonly used phrase in oriental medicine: 'Treatment is diagnosis and diagnosis is treatment.' In this respect, as will be seen in the next chapter, the basic approach of Western medicine is radically different from its Eastern counterpart.

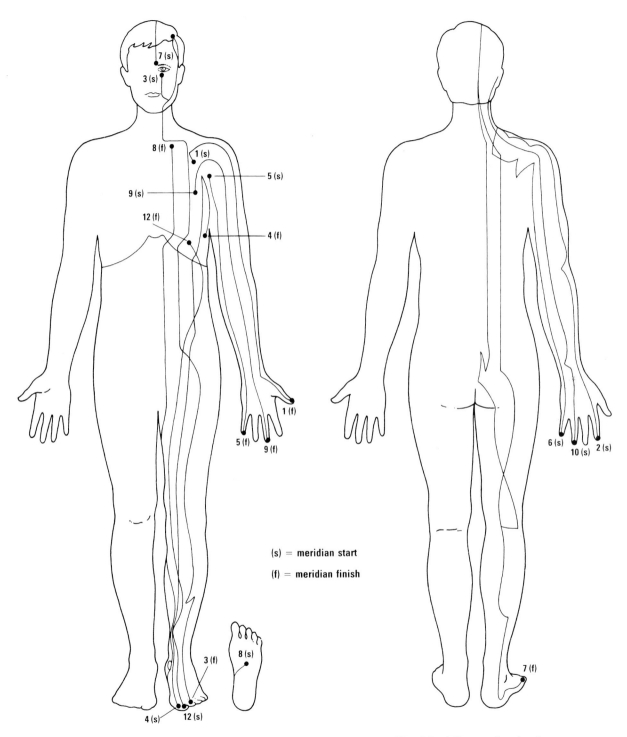

7 (s)

3 (s)

8 (f)

1 (s)

5 (s)

9 (s)

12 (f)

4 (f)

1 (f)

5 (f)

9 (f)

6 (s)

10 (s)

2 (s)

(s) = meridian start

(f) = meridian finish

3 (f)

8 (s)

7 (f)

4 (s)

12 (s)

The Meridians : front view

The Meridians : back view

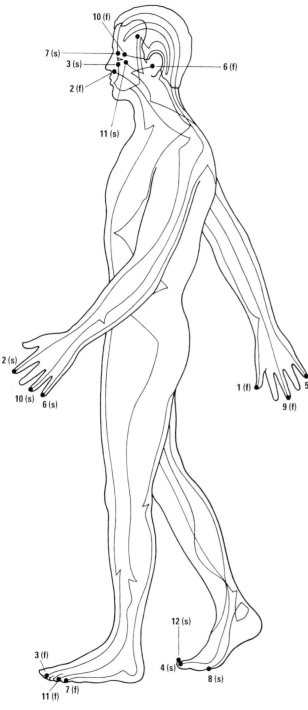

The Meridians : side view

KEY

All meridians are bilateral, meaning they appear symmetrically on both sides of the body. Only one side is shown on the front and back diagrams.

Meridians are numbered from 1–12 according to the flow of energy through them. (See energy flow through the meridians chart on page 15.)

All meridians start or finish in the head, chest, hands or feet.

1. **Lung** – Starts on chest in front of shoulder, finishes in thumb

2. **Large Intestine** – Starts in index finger, finishes at side of nostril

3. **Stomach** – Starts under eye, finishes in second toe

4. **Spleen** – Starts in big toe, finishes at side of chest

5. **Heart** – Starts under armpit, finishes in little finger

6. **Small Intestine** – Starts in little finger, finishes in front of ear

7. **Urinary Bladder** – Starts at inside corner of eye, finishes in little toe

8. **Kidney** – Starts on sole of foot, finishes at top of chest

9. **Heart Constrictor** – Starts beside nipple, finishes in middle finger

10. **Triple Heater** – Starts in fourth finger, finishes by outside corner of eyebrow

11. **Gall Bladder** – Starts at outside corner of eye, finishes in fourth toe

12. **Liver** – Starts in big toe, finishes on front of chest below nipple

The Benefits of Shiatsu

HEALTH, DISEASE, PREVENTION AND CURE

In the ancient medical classics of both East and West, health was defined as a function of one's ability to live in harmony with one's environment. This involved becoming highly sensitive to one's physical, mental and emotional patterns as well as to those of one's environment, and trying to balance them all out. In practice, as the orientals were quick to observe in their description of Yin and Yang, the universe and all creation are constantly changing. Staying healthy could therefore become a full-time occupation.

In fact, this is not far from the truth. Early oriental health practices, as I have mentioned, concentrated on staying healthy, and this certainly involved daily practice of some sort or another. This kind of activity often takes patience and commitment and is not easy to achieve. But classical texts talk of the natural lifespan as being at least a hundred years, and we ourselves still use the old biblical saying 'three score years and ten'. This begs the question: why are people dying so young these days? Yet modern medicine has produced so many apparent 'cures', especially for epidemic disease. Infant mortality rates are lower than ever in most parts of the world. If health really is measured in terms of the absence of disease, as modern medicine claims, then what of the quality and length of life itself? In this simple respect, the principles and practice of modern medicine compared with those of more traditional systems of both East and West could not be more different.

The concepts of 'medicine' and 'cure' are intrinsically alien to the oriental approach to health. The original role of the Eastern medical expert was to guide a person in health rather than to treat them for a disease. As the Yellow Emperor says: '... the sages did not treat those who were already ill; they instructed those who were not yet ill. They did not want to rule those who were already rebellious; they guided those who were not yet rebellious.' Naturally times have changed and today's stressful, polluted city lifestyle prevents many people from realistically following the example of the 'sages'. Nevertheless, oriental medicine as such still retains a strong slant towards prevention rather than intervention, and Shiatsu certainly fits this mould.

DIAGNOSIS AND TREATMENT

The Eastern tendency to consider the general before the particular is quite clearly evident in the oriental approach to health and health-care. Specific symptoms are rarely considered individually, but are seen instead to point to a wider picture of general body imbalance. The guiding principles of Yin and Yang and the many correspondences of the five transformations provide the means of painting this picture. Instead of reducing a given set of symptoms down to an isolated, definable cause, as in modern Western medicine, the oriental approach expands them into broader correspondences which allow a richer contrast to reveal the basic pattern of imbalance. When you focus directly on an object at night it becomes very hard to see it – in order to pick it out you must look obliquely at it and widen your field of vision.

Diagnosis as such, at least in the Western medical sense, does not apply to Shiatsu. Nor does the word 'treatment'. First, the Shiatsu practitioner cannot rely on any machines but must learn to trust the senses. Observing, listening, smelling, asking and, of course, touching are the main methods (usually referred to as the 'four methods') by which information is obtained. But logic does not determine the gathering of this information, and a Shiatsu 'diagnosis' relies on the practitioner's ability to remain alert, sensitive and non-judgemental throughout. This means registering information as it is perceived, by whatever means (verbal, auditory, visual or tactile), but not interpreting it. This is the basic paradox of oriental medicine, since the realm of 'diagnosis' collapses into the realm of 'treatment', and what is left can only be described as an interaction between giver and receiver during which information is constantly being evaluated and exchanged. Perhaps compassion and sympathy for the sick person are the only 'given' in this diagnosis/treatment equation.

However, it would be wrong to think that giving Shiatsu is like a shot in the dark. The Yin/Yang, five transformations and four methods models are designed to guide the practitioner to identify the nature, location and depth of a particular imbalance in a person's energy system, as we have seen. The sheer variety of possible approaches to any such imbalance, coupled with the basic benign effect of Shiatsu, ensures a measure of success even if the approach is off-course. Naturally, however, the clearer the picture becomes the more effective the outcome of any 'treatment' will be, and this fact cannot be avoided. What distinguishes professional Shiatsu from relaxation therapy is this ability to produce consistent results regardless of the methods of diagnosis or treatment. This book is just a beginning aimed at teaching some simple techniques of Shiatsu, and the ability to make someone feel good should not be confused with correcting specific imbalances in the mind and body.

EFFECTS

The main principle of treatment relied upon in Shiatsu is that of the body's own innate ability to balance and heal itself. The method by which this is achieved relies on the proper stimulation of the body's energy system which, as we have seen, includes the meridians and points. In practice, when correct pressure is applied (see the following chapter for principles of pressure) a positive effect is always achieved. That is to say the receiver's homeostatic or self-regulating abilities are activated and the system will begin to balance itself naturally. As mentioned in the chapter on the principles of Shiatsu, a 'Kyo' type person who is basically weaker will respond more slowly to this process than a 'Jitsu' type who is basically stronger. The job of the Shiatsu practitioner is to assess these strengths and weaknesses in terms of the person's illness and in their ability to respond to it and to redistribute their available energy resources to restore harmony to the system using the meridians.

Stimulation of the meridians and points frees up blocked energy and draws it towards areas of weakness. According to one of the laws of Yin and Yang discussed earlier, an extreme of one can transform to its opposite. So in areas of blockage (Jitsu) where there may be Yang phenomenon such as tightness, heat and pain which feels uncomfortable to the touch, firmer, quicker pressure (also Yang) is used to disperse the blockage – Yang meets Yang and turns to Yin producing release and relaxation. Conversely, in areas of weakness (Kyo) where there may be more Yin phenomena such as emptiness, cold and aches, which welcome touch, softer, lingering pressure (more Yin) may be used to draw energy to the area – Yin meets Yin and turns to Yang, producing an invigorating, revitalising effect.

These are basically the two main approaches to giving Shiatsu – the one more dynamic and releasing, the other more gentle and nourishing. The elements of stretch and manipulation shown in this book obviously relate to the former, whilst the latter include the more static pressure techniques. But within any one technique you can bring both Yin and Yang elements into play, and most Shiatsu is a natural combination of these. In practice, though, the type of Shiatsu shown in this book relies more on locating the weaker areas and working to nourish them by 'calling' the energy from other, more blocked areas. It is characterised therefore by quite a soft, gentle, smooth-flowing quality which requires you simply to rest or lean, not actively to 'do' anything, which is why it is sometimes referred to as 'Zen Shiatsu' or 'do nothing Shiatsu'.

In trying to describe the benefits of Shiatsu, I have avoided listing specific results in terms of the systems of the body as we understand them from a Western perspective. The fact is that Shiatsu does not lend itself well to this approach; and, unlike Western massage which has been adopted for its specific remedial effects in cases of tension, injury and so on, Shiatsu must be evaluated in terms of the system to which it belongs.

Attempts have been made to equate the oriental concept of the energy system with, for example, the nervous system, but these correspondences are imprecise and ultimately invalid. Naturally, since Shiatsu works on the body it affects the nervous, circulatory, respiratory and musculo-skeletal systems. However, through its stimulation of the hormone system it can also affect the digestive and reproductive systems. In fact, the more specific one attempts to be in describing the effects of Shiatsu, the more general and wide-reaching seems to be the picture.

It is interesting and perhaps not entirely coincidental that in another, related, field – that of modern physics – scientists have sought to define matter in the same reductionist way in which medicine has tried to define and treat the body. Yet the very latest research seems to have unearthed a fundamental paradox in this approach to knowledge – that the more you seek to reduce and define things into smaller and smaller parts in order to understand the whole, the more the whole seems to be implied in them in the first place. In fact, some of the leading modern physicists are engaged in dialogue with leading figures in the world of metaphysics, in order to investigate similarities in understanding energy and matter.

In the meantime, it is enough to say that Shiatsu can and does help with a variety of ailments, particularly chronic, persistent ones. Apart from bringing relief to symptoms, it gradually corrects long-term postural and behavioural imbalances leading to improved body/ mind awareness and a general sense of wellbeing and peace of mind. It is the purpose of Shiatsu to regulate the energetic system linking mind, body and spirit, and, as some scientists now seem ready to accept, perhaps the relationship between energy and matter can be explored intuitively just as well as with a rational, thinking approach. Perhaps the energetic model used by the orientals to understand and treat the body is more closely linked with the structural approach of modern medicine than we might think. It may not be long before the paradigm of scientific medicine expands to include such approaches as Shiatsu, acupuncture and many other forms of ener-getic medicine.

The Techniques of Shiatsu

NATURAL MOVEMENT AND PRESSURE

Shiatsu involves the application of static pressure to the body and is governed by the basic laws of physics. Gravity is our main ally, not our muscles, and the most important principle, universally applied to all techniques in Shiatsu, is that of natural, leaning pressure. Only the body weight is used, without pushing, pressing or squeezing, like a crawling baby whose body is supported without effort by its arms and legs. This may sound easy, and it certainly requires no effort, but in practice it often involves rediscovering the kind of unconscious, automatic and highly integrated way in which we first began using our bodies as babies. Of course you will improve with practice, and you don't have to be a dancer or an acrobat to do Shiatsu, but you must first learn the basics of *how* to apply pressure rather than *where*. This involves the careful positioning of your body so that you can lean or 'rest' on your partner, from any angle, in any position, comfortably and without effort.

Initially, then, learning Shiatsu involves practising and perfecting the art of moving into precisely the correct position to apply natural leaning pressure to any given area of the body. Such movements assume a rhythm and flow of their own, in which precision and grace, discipline and spontaneity combine in a dance-like sequence. This is often referred to as the 'form', and the purpose of this chapter is to highlight the importance of the principles of pressure which guide such a 'form'. As a beginner, it is far more effective to concentrate on learning to give good-quality pressure rather than trying to work out where to press next.

THE 'FORM'

All martial arts practitioners are familiar with the concept and practice of a particular 'form' of movement associated with their chosen discipline, be it Karate, Judo, Tai Chi or any other. In fact, this notion of 'form' extends to the study and practice of all oriental arts and sciences, from calligraphy to flower arranging, from the tea ceremony to paper folding. Indeed, a broader understanding of oriental culture in general reveals many subtle levels at which this concept of 'form' operates. The way one looks, behaves and even thinks are all greatly influenced by how these factors may appear to others. Conformity is considered a virtue and contributes to the collective 'form' of society and ultimately to its peace and harmony. To act out of self-interest shows disregard for the group and goes against the common good. In the field of medicine, to threaten such harmony (in this case symbolised by the accepted laws of nature) would be literally to endanger your health. Many of the medical classics emphasised the need to live in harmony with such laws, which governed all aspects of life including exercise, rest, diet, emotions and relationships as well as climate, season and geography.

Thus a concern for the 'form' of things is paramount, though this is not to say that such a concern is for things simply to look good – it has a purpose which is both subtle and powerful. It aims to liberate the mind and allow the body to experience things directly. For example, in Zen meditation there is a 'form' of sitting and walking while focusing on the breath, and maintaining a certain posture for a certain length of time. The ultimate purpose may be to attain a spiritual goal (enlightenment), but the 'form' is essentially practical. The more you concentrate on sitting, walking and breathing the less your mind tries to work out the purpose of it all. Only when the mind is quiet can the value of the experience of meditation be fully appreciated. What may at first seem empty ritual actually provides the focus for developing concentration, awareness and ultimately peace of mind.

In Shiatsu, the 'form' consists of a series of interconnected movements to enable the giver to apply correct leaning pressure to the different parts of the receiver's body. It requires a level of precision and skill which seem almost mechanical at first, but which, like the Zen example above, encourage concentration and quieten the mind to allow the direct experience of giving and receiving the pressure to be felt. Through the 'form' you will develop a level of body awareness and sensitivity which will far outweigh your ability to understand what it is you actually feel or do in Shiatsu. Curiously, perhaps, it is through the discipline of strict technical application that intuition, one of the key elements of Shiatsu, seems to develop. The 'form', once learnt, can become a liberating rather than a limiting experience.

The 'form' illustrated in this book is designed to give you access to the basic principles of Shiatsu and to allow you to practise a total body treatment in the prone and supine positions. The techniques shown are by no means a definitive sequence, but are part of a wide variety of movements that can be used to apply pressure to different parts of the body. In practice, of course, someone experienced in giving Shiatsu will select elements of the total 'form' in order to emphasise the areas selected for treatment. These will vary according to the diagnosis of energy imbalance in that person.

PRINCIPLES OF PRESSURE

These are the specific principles which govern the practice of Shiatsu and the actual techniques of applying the pressure.

1. Vertical Pressure

In order to apply natural leaning pressure when giving Shiatsu, the part of our body supporting our weight must be perpendicular to the surface being worked on. Since the human body has an eneven, undulating surface the angle of pressure must be adapted to each area in turn in order to maintain vertical pressure. In other words, we must always apply pressure towards the centre of any given part of the body as we work on it.

Pressure which is not perpendicular will become unsteady and often cause discomfort to the receiver.

2. Stationary Pressure

Static pressure is one of the main features which distinguishes Shiatsu from other massage forms. The pressure is held steadily at each point in turn, and is applied and released vertically in between moves. There is no rubbing, rotating, kneading or squeezing. The pressure is simply held in position for variable lengths of time, depending on how relaxing or invigorating you want the effect to be. Generally speaking, shorter, quicker movements are more stimulating than slow, patient pressure held for a long time, which is very calming. Often it is best to follow your partner's breathing, applying the pressure as they breathe out and releasing again as they inhale.

Pressure which is unstable and shaky will cause too much stimulation to your partner's nervous system, and their body will be unable to relax fully and receive all the benefits of deep, penetrating pressure.

3. Supporting Pressure

When we are sitting in a comfortable chair, for the most part we are not conscious of the job the chair is doing to support us. The same is true of our muscles, some of which are working to maintain our position even though we are unaware of it most of the time. Only when we move do we momentarily become aware of the need to direct our bodies into the new position and support them there. The subtle, supportive quality of this type of relationship is what we are aiming at when we apply pressure in Shiatsu. We want our partner to feel completely supported, physically and emotionally, by our actions. The way we handle their body needs to convey trust and a feeling of security, so that they can 'switch off' to what we are actually doing and their body can relax completely. In practical terms, this involves paying careful attention to the 'support' hand (or elbow/knee), which acts as a base for our body weight and also firmly keeps our partner in a stable position. Meanwhile, the 'giving' hand (or elbow/knee) can get on with giving the pressure. When both hands are working together (for example on the face), part of the contact area on each hand does the job of supporting while the thumbs give the pressure. These aspects are stressed in the captions accompanying the photographs in this book.

Pressure which is not supportive will not allow you to give proper vertical and stationary pressure – and, more importantly, will not allow your partner to relax. The partner will tend to try and 'help' you do the movements, and the effect of your pressure will be minimised.

4. *Equal Pressure*

The importance of equal pressure is closely linked to that of supporting pressure (see above). For the nervous system to relax completely, and for your partner to begin to loosen and open up to your pressure, that pressure needs to be both supportive and equal. That is to say that the amount of pressure applied to all areas of contact, whether supporting or giving, must be equal. Naturally, as you shift from one position to another your pressure will momentarily be unequal, but the important thing is to equalise it again as soon as possible. The effect is to enhance the quality of supportiveness and help relax your partner further, just as when you lie on your bed the constant, equal pressure exerted by the mattress against your body supports and relaxes you.

Pressure which is not equal feels sharp and invasive and will prevent your partner relaxing deeply during the Shiatsu, partly because they will be more conscious of what you are doing and partly because your pressure will not penetrate so deeply.

TECHNIQUES OF PRESSURE

As this is essentially designed as a workbook, I have placed a lot of emphasis on the practical, step-by-step application of pressure using the 'form' or integrated sequence illustrated in the photographs. I hope that from these you will be able to observe clearly the appropriate body positioning and correct application of pressure in each individual sequence, and that the accompanying captions will clarify the movements where necessary.

In terms of the actual techniques used to apply the active pressure, you will notice that I use the elbows quite a lot. This brings you into closer contact with your partner and provides you with a wider area of support for your body weight. However, it takes some time to develop sensitivity here, as it does in the knees, and at the beginning I suggest you experiment with your hands, which are generally more sensitive and less likely to cause pain or discomfort to your partner. Most of the sequences shown using the elbows can easily be performed with the hands instead as long as the basic principles of pressure (page 24) are closely observed. Shiatsu is a flexible and dynamic treatment, and almost any part of the body can be used effectively to apply pressure. On the opposite page are the parts of the body used at one time or another in this book. In the meantime here are some points to remember when studying the sequences in this book:

1. The exact positioning shown for each technique is comfortable for me. If your body size is radically different or you are left-handed or need to compensate in some other way, try to adjust your body position accordingly, bearing in mind the basic principles of applying the pressure.

2. Concentrate on getting your techniques right *before* you try to match them up with the meridian diagrams. Don't try to work on specific meridians until you are comfortable with your 'form' and fluent at it.

3. Start with the easier techniques first so as to gain confidence, and in the beginning use your thumbs and palms more than any parts of the body as they are more sensitive than the elbows or knees and less likely to cause discomfort to your partner.

4. Pay as much attention to the overall flow of your movements as to each individual sequence. Practise the whole 'form' right through until it becomes automatic and you don't have to think about each movement before you do it.

5. At the same time as concentrating on technique, try not to do this at the expense of losing an overall sense of purpose in your work. In other words, remember that you are trying to make your partner feel good and that the quality of your Shiatsu depends as much on your overall approach as on specific techniques.

1. THUMBS

In some forms of Shiatsu, thumb pressure is the most commonly used technique. In this book I have used it to apply pressure to small, precise areas like bone crevices, in between muscles and on certain specific 'acupoints'. These include the head, face, neck, hands, feet and sacrum.

The thumbs should not be bent but should make a straight, continuous line with the forearm. Use the area between the tip and the ball of the thumb to apply the pressure. Equal and supporting pressure is given by the insides of the fingers, so that the thumbs themselves do not feel too invasive. Thumb pressure can easily become tiring and you may need to do regular exercises to strengthen them.

2. FINGERS

The fingers are mainly used in a supportive role for thumb or palm Shiatsu, but can be used for grasping techniques when a whole area, such as the arm, is pressed at once. They are also used to give pressure on the chest but are otherwise reserved for abdominal palpation, principally to take a diagnosis (not shown in this book).

3. PALMS

Probably the most widely used part of the body in Shiatsu, the palms are very sensitive and can be used to mould themselves to a wide area of your partner's body. This means you can apply quite a lot of pressure, without causing discomfort, to curved areas like the arms and legs as well as to flatter areas like the back. The heel of the palm can be used to give more precise pressure, though in this book I have mostly used it to give general, overall pressure to prepare areas as well as to go over them at the end of a sequence.

4. ELBOWS

More precisely it is an area on the forearm just below the elbow that is used, rather than the point of the elbow itself. The point often gives too strong, focused pressure and can easily cause discomfort. This technique is mainly used for large, muscular areas such as the back, legs and buttocks, where pressure can be fairly deep and strong without causing discomfort. It may take time to get used to this technique and to develop sensitivity in that part of your body, but it is a very useful and relaxing way to give Shiatsu and I have demonstrated it a lot in this book.

5. KNEES

Despite their power and size, the knees can give very soft, relaxing pressure, partly because your body weight is spread over a large area and partly because you use both hands to give support, giving three areas of contact altogether. This makes equal pressure more difficult to maintain as you have three separate points to equalise.

Take care in applying pressure with the knees since they lack sensitivity and, like the elbows, it is harder to gauge the correct amount of pressure to apply. The knees are mainly used on large, soft areas like the legs and sometimes the arms.

6. FEET

The feet are highly sensitive areas of our body. They carry our entire weight most of the time, and form our direct link with the ground beneath. They are used extensively in many massage forms, especially in Indian massage, some of which is done entirely with the feet. The original form of Shiatsu was probably 'barefoot', where the body was literally walked all over from head to foot. I have included walking on the back of the thighs and the soles of the feet in this book, though in fact almost any part of the body can be pressed by the feet. It is, however, a technique that requires good balance and coordination if it is to be done safely, and you shouldn't experiment unsupervised.

In practice, a combination of all these techniques is used. Common to them all is the use of the basic principles described in this chapter, which govern every technique of Shiatsu. Added to these pure techniques are the proper use of the 'Hara' and the breath, which will be described in the following chapter.

Preparing to Give and Receive Shiatsu

NOTE TO THE RECEIVER

This chapter is aimed primarily at the giver of Shiatsu, though as a receiver you can benefit from all the preparatory points mentioned here. For example, you are likely to get more out of your Shiatsu in the long term if you take regular exercise and do some form of relaxation. Shiatsu is a two-way process and relies to some extent on the responsiveness of the receiver as well as the giver. When receiving Shiatsu you will often be expected to participate actively in the treatment by using your breath to relax your whole body, and in between sessions by following a series of exercises designed to enhance the therapeutic effect. Essentially, Shiatsu works best when it is able to impact the various factors which affect your overall health, and this naturally extends beyond the treatment time itself. This in turn requires a certain level of commitment on your part.

ENVIRONMENT

Choose a room that is quiet, clean and tidy, with as few distractions as possible and a pleasant 'feel' to it. Natural light is preferable, though it should not be too bright, and fresh air is essential. Ideally there should be as little noise as possible, and though some people may like background music to relax them initially this can be turned off once you begin the Shiatsu – indeed, it may be distracting. The room temperature should be comfortable but not stuffy; you should have a blanket nearby for particularly cold people and for covering your partner at the end of the treatment.

   You want your partner to feel comfortable in every respect, but not so much so that they switch off to their surroundings and to you. The ideal state to be in when receiving Shaitsu is somewhere between being awake and asleep, in a state of complete relaxation as in meditation. In this state you are more deeply relaxed, in fact, than when simply asleep, and you are much more receptive to the Shiatsu.

TIME AND FREQUENCY OF TREATMENT

Shiatsu can be done at any time of the day, though according to the theory of energy circulation and season there is always an ideal time for each individual. Since the techniques shown in this book are for beginners and your Shiatsu is likely to be used mainly for general relaxation purposes, the evening would be an ideal time for you to give a Shiatsu before your partner goes to bed. On the other hand, Shiatsu can be very invigorating and the early morning is also a good time to choose. In any event, never give Shiatsu when you or your partner are over-tired, still digesting a meal, or under the influence of alcohol.

Where possible, allow your partner to rest for about fifteen minutes following the treatment and make sure they are covered with a blanket as the body often gets cold after a long period of inactivity. Stay in the room, as they may 'come to' and momentarily be disorientated – but they will be reassured by your presence. Never give much more than an hour's Shiatsu at one time; if you do, the effects can often be counter-productive. It seems that the body has a sort of 'attention span' rather like the mind, and this varies from person to person. In some cases thirty minutes will be enough.

It is perfectly healthy to receive up to two or even three Shiatsu treatments a week, though in practice one is usual. If you are working on a specific problem, such as a stiff neck, you will need to do a series of treatments to make a lasting difference, though the first time a person receives Shiatsu is often the most dramatic.

EQUIPMENT

Shiatsu is always given on floor level, usually on the kind of Japanese cotton mattress known as a futon. Alternatively use any foam mattress or blanket that is fairly firm and not springy – a sprung mattress is no good. Your partner must be supported properly as you apply your weight, which is why a bed is not suitable. The floor is better than a treatment couch, as you can move around your partner much more easily and can lean your body weight over the top of them without effort. If a pillow is used (in the supine position) it should be firm and small; an ordinary bed pillow is not usually appropriate. The giver and receiver should both wear loose, natural-fibre (cotton) clothing – a thin tracksuit is fine (but make sure you wear one without zips!). When giving Shiatsu to areas of exposed skin such as the hands, feet, face and neck, a thin cotton hand towel or cloth can be used if you find it convenient. Unlike in other massage forms, we do not generally make direct contact with the bare skin in Shiatsu, since we neither apply anything to it (like oils) nor do we need to slide along it. The thin layer of cotton between the giver and receiver allows the giver to move easily from one position to the next without stretching or pinching the skin, and avoids any unpleasant contact if the giver or receiver has cold, sweaty or clammy skin.

CONTRA-INDICATIONS

The basic guidelines as to when and where not to give or receive Shiatsu are similar to those of any treatment which affects the flow of energy, blood and body fluids through the system. These would include times of high fever, especially when accompanied by local infection or inflammation or by infectious disease of any sort; cancer; heart disease; and areas where there may be cuts, bruises, scar tissue, injury or swelling.

However, since Shiatsu techniques vary from the very dynamic to the soft and gentle, it could still be possible to use the supportive quality of some of the holding techniques (see the previous chapter) in most of these situations. In fact, Shiatsu has been used effectively to complement other approaches in the treatment of various forms of cancer, heart disease, HIV + and AIDS.

For the purposes of this book, use your common sense and don't try any of the more dynamic movements on old, frail or weak-boned people; and don't give Shiatsu to anyone whom you are not confident in treating. It takes many years to qualify as a Shiatsu 'practitioner', and the sequences in this book are designed mainly to teach you to give Shiatsu for relaxation.

'HARA' AND THE BREATH

In Western medicine the brain is considered the single most vital organ, and we define death by its failure. The abdomen, by contrast, is rather a poor relation – merely the soft shell protecting the so-called 'vital' organs which, these days, can be removed or replaced with apparent ease and without major threat to life. Why then should oriental medicine, art and culture make such a fuss, as they do, about 'Hara'? This Japanese word basically means 'belly' or 'abdomen', yet what it embraces is much greater than that. The concept is an all-pervasive social and cultural one in the East, rooted in the earliest metaphysical and later medical writings. In the *Dao De Jing* by Lao Tsu it says that 'the Chinese sage becomes the abdomen (puts his consciousness in his abdomen). He doesn't become his eyes (put his consciousness in his sense perceptions).' This suggests that 'Hara' embodies a kind of sixth sense which incorporates and exceeds the other five.

In an early oriental classic, *Difficult Questions*, constant reference is made to the abdomen as being 'the source of the vital energies' from which the whole person is nourished. It is described as the 'root origin of the twelve meridians ... and the gate of breathing', hence the emphasis on the breath in Eastern preventative medicine, meditation and treatment. The abdomen is likened to the roots of a tree which, when properly nourished, in turn nourish the stems and branches (meridians and organs) to maintain good health and restore balance to the system.

In early medical literature, therefore, the abdomen was clearly accepted as the physical and spiritual centre of the body. In the martial arts, from which the basic theories of oriental medicine are drawn, movement 'from the centre' is considered the single most important discipline to master; it involves the integration of mental and physical skills, as in Shiatsu. Indeed the ultimate aim of all martial arts, as well as of other art forms like the tea ceremony, calligraphy and of course medicine, is to become a more rounded, 'centred' human being – to lose oneself in the practice, and yet to gain strength and understanding through it.

Interestingly, the phrase for an open-hearted or open-minded person in Japanese is *Hara ga okii desu*, which literally means they have a 'big Hara'. Amongst the many Buddhas the one with the biggest belly, usually sitting and always happy and content, is known as the laughing Buddha, as if a big 'Hara' both literally and symbolically suggests happiness and peace of mind.

Certainly the 'Hara' is a symbol of mind and body united, and to focus one's energies there is to seek to understand and develop oneself fully and completely. 'Hara kiri', literally meaning to 'cut the Hara', signifies the Japanese ritual form of suicide, since by this action the person is literally tearing out their centre, that vital part which defines them and gives them life.

In the West, we do have the concept of 'centredness', but it is usually something we conceive of intellectually. This separation of mind and body is completely alien to the concept and practice of 'Hara'. Some of us may trust our 'gut feeling', but we essentially distinguish this from pure thought. 'Hara' describes thought, feeling and action as a unified experience. To be good at something technically, without the intention and committedness from within, would be considered empty or hollow – there is no 'Hara' to inspire it and give it depth. Similarly, to show inspiration without proficient technique to put it into practice would be considered vain and capricious – no 'Hara' to ground it. This appreciation of 'Hara' permeates all aspects of life in oriental societies and is particularly strongly developed in the healing arts.

Thus in Shiatsu we must learn to integrate technique with understanding, and theory with practice, in order to develop 'Hara' as our physical and energetic centre. This can only be done through practice and should include a variety of approaches including Shiatsu itself, exercise and meditation. It must be experienced by the individual and cannot be taught. Essentially it is 'Hara' that makes the difference between Shiatsu being purely an effective manipulative tool and becoming a powerful healing therapy for both giver and receiver.

EXERCISE AND MEDITATION

The role of exercise and meditation is vital to the enjoyment and practice of Shiatsu. If you are not basically fit and lack patience and concentration, you will find Shiatsu difficult – though not impossible – to do. Since the aim of Shiatsu therapy is to maintain and restore the health of others, those giving it must themselves be examples of good health. In one of the oldest classics of oriental medicine, *The Yellow Emperor's Classic of Internal Medicine*, it says that 'those who are habitually without disease help to train and adjust those who are sick, for those who treat should be free from illness ... and in order to train the patient, they act as examples'. Quite a tall order! Nevertheless, the basic truth remains the same: the healthier you are, the easier and more effective your Shiatsu is likely to be.

Through regular exercise, anyone can develop the flexibility, balance, coordination, awareness, strength and fitness necessary for giving Shiatsu. Similarly, through meditation of any kind the mind can be trained to become focused, alert and calm, and to free itself from the confusions and stresses of a busy lifestyle. Meditation itself is intensely personal and may be done as effectively in the bath or on a mountain as in a church, synagogue, mosque or temple. Some people like chants or music, others complete silence. Some may lie or sit cross-legged, while others kneel or even stand. Some seem able to meditate anywhere, any time. In all schools of meditation, though, the essential purpose is the same: to allow the mind to calm itself, thoughts to subside, and a genuine sense of inner peace to fill our mind and body. The practice of meditation brings discipline and clarity to Shiatsu and also helps reveal and develop its more intuitive aspects.

On a more physical level, exercise is an essential part of improving our effectiveness at giving Shiatsu. It is hard to give proper pressure when our bodies are inflexible, as we cannot position ourselves correctly without feeling awkward and uncomfortable. Since Shiatsu is done on the floor, the toes, ankles and knees especially need regular exercise, as of course do the hands and fingers in order to provide the level of flexibility needed to move freely and without effort. Just as an athlete would never go into competition without a warm-up or without having followed a careful training programme, so, when preparing to give Shiatsu, we must loosen up the whole body and in the long term take regular exercise to move the 'Ki', to keep the tendons and ligaments loose, the muscles flexible and strong and the joints mobile.

It is not within the scope of this book to show detailed exercises, but here are three very simple movements which, when combined, stretch and work the major muscle groups and meridian systems in the body and move the 'Hara' in three directions – to the side, front and back. Make sure you also include elements of stretch, aerobic, coordination and breathing exercises in other things you do, both in warming up and in the long term. You should always do at least a 10-minute warm-up before giving a Shiatsu treatment. If possible join a Tai Chi or yoga class, and combine this 'internal' exercise with more 'external' forms, such as swimming, which improve cardio-vascular fitness. You don't need to be super-fit to do Shiatsu – but it helps!

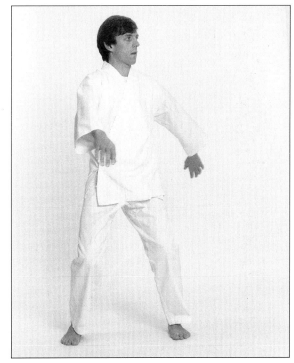

1. Side swing, see page 34

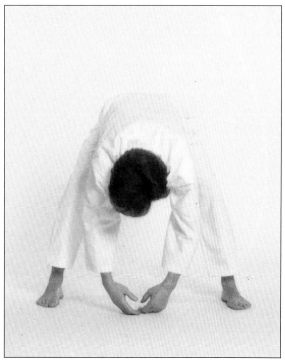

2. Forward and back rock, see page 34

SIDE SWING (1, page 33)

Stand with your feet shoulder-width apart, toes pointing forward. Bend your legs slightly at the knees. Begin turning to one side, using your hips and lower belly to guide the movement and letting your arms follow loosely. Allow this movement to gather momentum as you turn from side to side, keeping your arms loose, hips open and knees over the tops of your feet (don't let then collapse inwards). Keep the hips level, spine straight and chin tucked into the chest as you get a nice, smooth, relaxed rhythm going from side to side, loosening up the whole body.

FORWARD AND BACK ROCK (2, page 33)

The same start position as above, but this time with your feet slightly wider apart. Bend forward and down from the waist, letting your upper body and arms hang loosely towards the floor. Slowly begin rocking forward and back, so that as you go forward you reach back between your legs along the floor, and as you rock back you stretch up and reach back over your head. Control this movement from your hips with an undulating motion of the pelvis forward and back. Don't reach back too far, especially if you have a weak or sore back, but just allow the movement to flow freely and effortlessly. Keep your body as loose as possible.

SIDE STRETCH AND SWAY (3a and b)

This time, start with your feet even wider apart. Again bend forward and hang loosely down. Slowly begin to sway your whole upper body from side to side, trailing your hands along the floor. Increase the momentum of your swing until you make an arc from left to right and back again. As you reach each extremity of the arc, turn your body at the waist to face forwards. Hold this position momentarily before returning in an arc in the other direction. At the end of each swing, as you turn at the waist, you will stretch the whole side of your body and lift your arm over your head, looking up under the armpit.

When you are thoroughly warmed and loosened up, ask your partner to sit or lie in the position

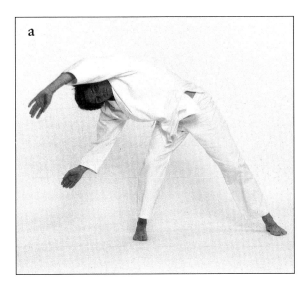

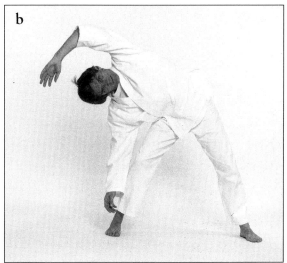

in which you wish to start giving your Shiatsu. The sequences in this book are designed for you to start with the sitting position and follow with the prone and supine positions. These are complete in themselves and each will give you enough techniques to provide at least thirty to forty minutes of Shiatsu. The sitting position sequences are preparatory warm-ups to loosen your partner up and will only take about ten minutes. Once you get used to doing the whole 'form' from start to finish you should complete the entire treatment in about an hour.

THE SITTING POSITION

This position has a number of advantages as well as one or two things to be aware of. It can be used as a warm-up before getting your partner to lie down and beginning a full body treatment or, for busy people with only a few minutes to spare, it can provide some welcome on-the-spot attention. In either case it can be done virtually anywhere, any time, since you can successfully perform most of the movements equally well on the floor or in a chair.

If you treat in a chair, use a straight-backed one with no arms so that your partner's back remains as straight as possible and is well supported. Make sure the height is right for you to be able comfortably to lean over your partner without standing on tiptoe.

If you work at floor level, have your partner sit in the most comfortable position for them, which is usually with the legs crossed. In the absence of chair support you must be careful to use your own body as support to keep them comfortable in the upright position. In other words *support* is the key word in this position, as your partner must feel able to relax completely whilst sitting otherwise they will tense their back muscles to keep themselves upright and this will defeat the object of the treatment. Don't keep them sitting up for too long, either, as this is not a relaxing enough position to maintain for long.

THE BENEFITS

In a full-body Shiatsu treatment the sitting position may or may not be used by the practitioner, but in any case would almost certainly be included near the beginning as a preparatory position. It can be used very effectively as a quick 'rub-down' for those all-important areas of tension in the head, neck and shoulders, and is excellent for upper body work in general including dynamic, opening chest/arm stretches. I have included here those elements of a more elaborate sitting sequence which I feel will help relax and prepare your partner for the following two positions. People often take a few minutes to 'arrive' and begin to unwind, and these few simple sequences will help get them used to your touch and allow you to get a first impression of their body – to feel the 'lie of the land', as it were. It is also a good time to exchange a little chat before the main part of the treatment, which is best done in silence. You only need spend ten minutes or so on these sequences before asking your partner to lie down on their front ready for the prone position.

FIRST CONTACT

The moment you first make physical contact with your partner is crucial to the whole treatment. It sets the tone and determines the quality of your work. With it you begin to become sensitive to your partner's tensions and weaknesses and therefore to their needs, whilst your partner begins to respond to your touch. The response you are aiming for is one of trust, so that with every movement their body will begin to relax and open up to you. This can be achieved directly by the quality of the first few moments of contact. It can take much longer if you don't give proper emphasis to this vital part of your treatment.

Don't attempt making contact until you feel completely relaxed and comfortable in your position. Ideally you will have done some preparatory exercises (see previous chapter) and will be feeling warm and loosened up. Sit with your legs tucked under (Japanese style), knees slightly apart, facing your partner's back, at about an arm's length from them. Keep your shoulders loose during the movement. Encourage your partner to trust you and let themselves be fully supported by you. You will do this by the gentle yet decisive quality of your movements.

THE BENEFITS

In palming down the spine, back and shoulders you are essentially gathering information rather than giving pressure for any specific result. You may notice tension or weakness in certain areas, which may differ from left to right; you can make a mental note of these for later. Your partner should feel properly supported and able to relax fully into the position. The main benefit of the first contact, then, is to reassure your partner and to give you hints as to where to focus your treatment later.

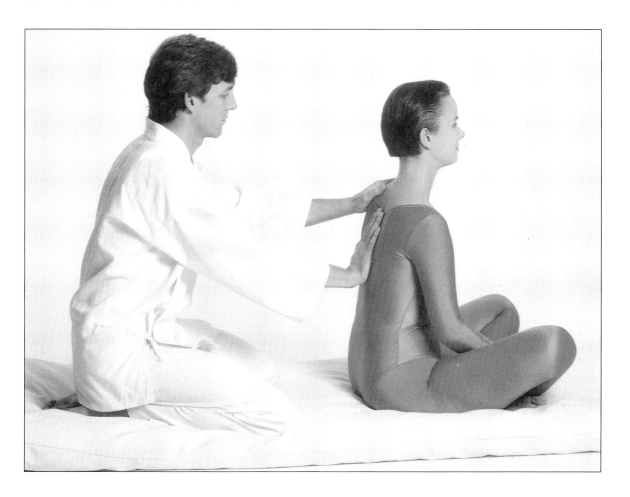

STEP 1 ▲
Lean forward from the hips, placing your left hand on your partner's left shoulder and gently easing their upper body towards you. At the same time extend the right arm forward, placing the palm over the spine in the area between the shoulder blades. Hold for several breaths, concentrating and 'tuning in' to your partner. Apply very gentle pressure to successive areas down the spine from top to bottom, using your left hand to support your partner.

STEP 2
Keep the left hand in the same position, moving your right palm to the left of your partner's spine, and give pressure in the same way down the muscle from top to bottom. Change hands, supporting with your right hand on their right shoulder and working down the right side of the spine on the muscle.

STEP 3
Finally 'wipe' down both sides of the spine together and then 'wipe' over and around the shoulder blades, giving the shoulders a gentle squeeze before moving on to the neck . . . .

Now move to a 45° angle behind and to the left side of your partner keeping one hand in contact with their back to support their body weight. Placing your left hand on their shoulder, lean forward to begin neck Shiatsu with the right hand . . . .

NECK/OCCIPUT PRESSURE

In giving pressure to the neck, the angle at which you sit is important. If you are directly behind your partner you will be unable to reach the side of the neck, whilst if you sit totally to one side you won't reach the back of the neck. But by sitting at a 45° angle behind and to the side of your partner you will be able to give pressure to all the areas of the neck without moving your position. Things to watch with this movement are that the angle of your pressure to the neck is kept perpendicular, and that you don't squeeze the neck with thumb and fingers – rather you lean in and apply pressure with a soft hand.

In giving pressure to the occiput (the base of the skull), make sure your partner's back is fully supported by the inside of your thigh and that they are comfortable. In applying the pressure, don't use your strength; simply bring the two hands together as if you were gently squeezing a balloon from either side. Don't tense the thumb or fingers.

In both sequences your intention should be to provide proper support to your partner, so that they can relax their neck and shoulders completely.

THE BENEFITS

A tremendous amount of tension is carried in the neck and occipital area – not least from the sheer weight of carrying our head around all the time! Referred tension and pain from the shoulders or upper back may also be reflected in the neck. Firm, penetrating pressure to these areas can provide great relief from tension and stiffness as well as alleviating pain. Headaches especially can be helped by these sequences, and particularly by pressure to the base and back of the skull.

In oriental medicine we focus here on the six Yang meridians which all begin or end in the head, concentrating especially on the gall bladder and urinary bladder for the relief of headaches. (See meridian drawings on pages 16 and 17.)

STEP 1 ▶

Begin with the left side of the neck (usually looser in right-handed people). Lean forward from the hips, placing your left hand on your partner's left shoulder, and gently easing them towards you. At the same time extend the right arm forward, cupping the neck in your palm, with the thumb on the near side and the fingers wrapped around the far side. Apply gentle thumb pressure to the neck along three lines (shown in the diagram) from the base of the skull downward. Use your body weight to lean in, holding your partner steady with your left hand. Keep your thumb and fingers soft – don't tense or squeeze them. (For clarity, this photograph shows Shiatsu to the right side of the neck.)

STEP 2 ▶

Step forward with your right foot, keeping the left knee on the ground, and kneel up to bring the inside of your right thigh and leg to support your partner's back. Transfer your support hand from your partner's shoulder to their forehead. Keep your right hand in the same position, sliding the thumb under the base of the skull and cupping the neck as before. Apply gentle pressure along the base of the skull from behind the ear to the nape of the neck (shown in the diagram). Press your hands towards each other, using equal pressure directed to the centre of the head. Don't tense your thumb.

Repeat Steps 1 and 2 on the other side. Then remain in position for the neck stretches and rotations . . . .

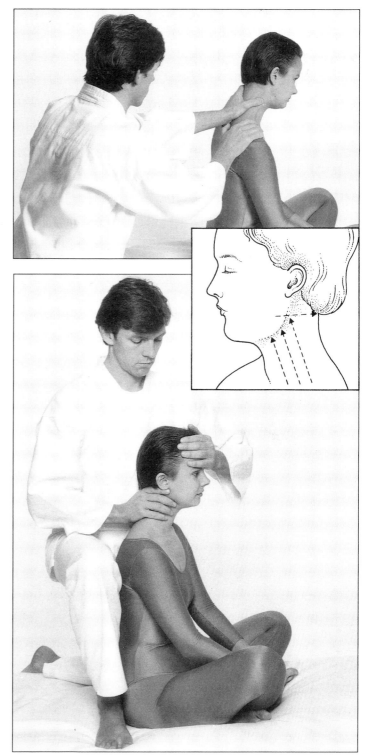

NECK STRETCHES/ROTATIONS

Shiatsu, though it focuses on the application of static pressure, includes elements of stretch and gentle manipulation. However, these are always performed following proper relaxing of the area to be stretched or manipulated. The basic rule, therefore, is pressure first, then stretch and finally manipulation.

In the following sequences it is vital that pressure to the neck is given before attempting to stretch or manipulate it. Rotating a stiff neck before loosening it adequately will cause it to stiffen further, and may be painful and even dangerous. When manipulating the neck you must make positive and decisive, though still very gentle, movements, encouraging your partner to relax completely and trust your guidance. If they try to help you with any of the movements – or, worse still, to resist you at all – you must abandon the sequence and return to it later. *Never* force any of these movements.

The main thing to concentrate on is a firm support hand, which should immobilise the neck and only allow the head to move around it.

If your partner has injured their neck or you are treating an elderly person, make small, gentle movements. When in doubt, leave these sequences out altogether.

THE BENEFITS

Performed properly, these stretches and manipulations are an excellent reinforcement of the neck and occiput pressure shown in the previous sequence. They help soften and loosen the whole neck and release tension in the muscles and meridians, relieving stiffness and pain and improving mobility. In Shiatsu, maintaining a balanced flow of energy in the meridians to and from the head is vital in order to avoid an excess of Yang building up in the upper body. Yang energy has a tendency to rise, and when blocked will cause heat, stiffness and pain.

STEP 1 ▶

Having finished giving pressure to the base of the skull on your partner's right side, maintain your position with your right hand supporting their forehead, and your left leg up supporting their back. Slide your left hand round to the left side of their neck to form a loose fist, tucking your knuckles under the base of their skull. Allow the back of your hand to rest on their shoulder and your forearm to rest on your knee. Then gently roll their head backwards on to your knuckles at a 45° angle, stretching it to its natural limit. Don't *force* the stretch – simply press your hands towards each other gently. (For clarity, this photograph shows Shiatsu to the left side of the neck.)

Change sides, mirroring your position, and repeat the movement to the right side of the neck.

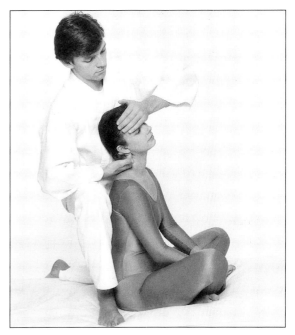

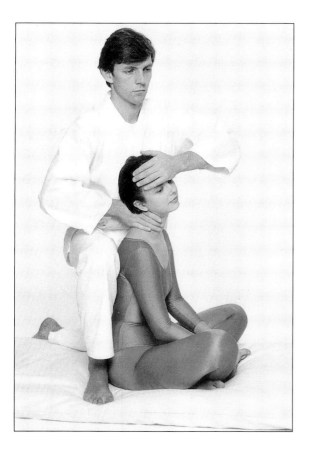

STEP 2 ◀

Having crossed over to your partner's left side to finish the right side neck stretch, maintain your position with your left hand supporting their forehead and your right leg up supporting their back. Uncurl your right fist and gently grasp their neck with your palm, thumb on the near side, fingers wrapped around the far side, tucking the knuckle of your forefinger under the base of the skull. Gently begin rotating the head, using your left hand to guide the movement whilst maintaining good support with the right. Begin with half rotations to the rear first. Then, if the neck feels loose enough, make full, flowing circles in both directions. *Never* force the movement.

Change sides, mirroring your position, and repeat the movement to the left side of the neck. End up where you began, on your partner's right side.

Now reach forward with your left hand to take hold of their left arm just above the elbow, and get ready to begin the arm rotations and shoulder stretches . . . .

ARM ROTATIONS/SHOULDER STRETCHES

Since there is a direct correspondence between the neck and the shoulders, in terms of both muscles and meridians, it is usual to work on the head, neck and shoulders as one whole area at the same time. So here we follow work on the neck with some stretching of the shoulder muscles and loosening of the joint. However, when you move an entire limb in Shiatsu – in this case the arm – there are several things to keep in mind.

Firstly, if your partner is heavily built and their arm is large, you will tire easily if you rely on your strength alone to move it. You must use your entire body – hands, arms, shoulders, torso and especially hips – to create momentum in the movement and to reduce the amount of effort you need to put in. This requires a combination of timing and balance, and has nothing to do with physical strength. No matter how small you are or how big your partner, if you use your body correctly you will be able to manipulate arms and even legs effortlessly!

Secondly, if your partner has trouble relaxing or their muscles are stiff or very developed, you will find they have a tendency either to help or to resist you in the movement. In other words, they cannot simply let you do the work. It is difficult to stretch and manipulate in these cases, but usually a quick shake of the arm will call their attention to the fact that they are not fully relaxed, and this may be enough to let you take control of the movement. Saying 'Just let your arm go heavy' may be effective. Don't say 'relax'!

In gauging the stretch, at first ask your partner how far to go. Gradually you will develop the sensitivity to do this without asking.

In manipulating the shoulder joint do not 'pull through' the joint – i.e. force it round in too large an arc.

Finally, make sure you give good support with the inside of your leg against their back, so as to keep their upper body stable.

THE BENEFITS

Stiff shoulders are a common problem and can be the cause of other ailments such as stiff neck, tension headaches and backache. These stretches can be very beneficial to the flexibility of the upper body.

In terms of the meridians, we can stretch the arm Yin meridians (Step 1) as well as the small intestine meridian (Step 2). By rotating the arm and shoulder we are mainly working on the small intestine meridian, which is distributed over the whole shoulder blade. Loosening the joint will have a balancing effect on the gall bladder meridian.

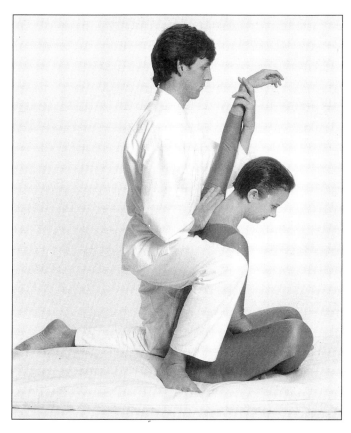

STEP 1 ◀

After the last neck rotation keep your right leg up, supporting your partner's back, and with your left hand take hold of their left arm just above the elbow. Slide your right hand across from the right side of their neck and place it on their left shoulder. Bring their arm up and rotate it gently a few times to check their flexibility. Then bring the arm up vertically to brush the side of the head, at the same time sliding your right palm down on to the shoulder blade and pressing forward, using your hips. You can vary the angle of the arm to stretch different muscles and meridians. The stretch is created by the 'push-me-pull-you' effect of your two hands moving in opposite directions. Again, the support hand on the shoulder blade does most of the work. *Don't* use your strength to pull their arm back, just lean.

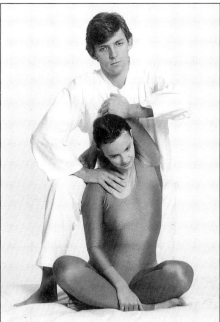

STEP 2 ◀

Now bring the arm up vertically, brushing the side of your partner's head. At the top of the arc allow the forearm to bend and flop down over the back of the head, supporting the upper arm just above the elbow with your left hand. Slide your right hand across from the left shoulder blade to the right side of your partner's neck. With both your elbows raised, press your hands gently together, stretching their arm over and behind their head, which will naturally drop forward. Make sure you keep their body upright.

Change sides, mirroring your position, and repeat both movements on the right side.

Release the left arm and let it flop down to your partner's side. Stand up behind your partner, letting them rest against your legs. Lean over and down, placing your palms on their shoulders ready for the shoulder pressure lift and drop . . . .

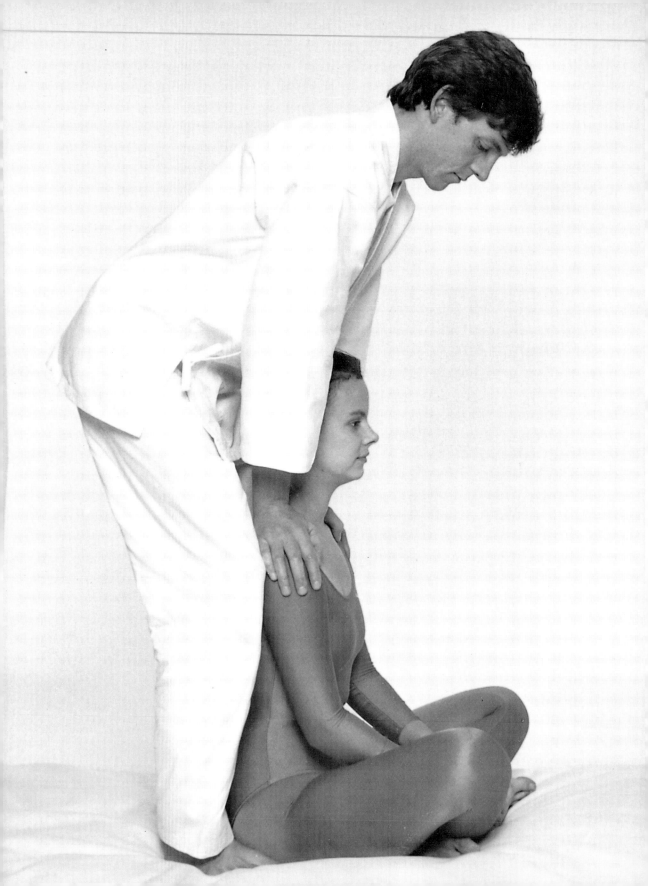

SHOULDER PRESSURE LIFT AND DROP

Any work on the head, neck and shoulders would be incomplete without pressure applied to the tops of the shoulders from above. You can work with the palms pressing down on the whole shoulder area, or be more specific with the thumbs getting into the large band of muscle across the back of the shoulders (the trapezius).

The advantage of standing above your partner is that you only have to lean your body weight gently forward and down to apply pressure without the need to push or to use muscle power. The more relaxed you are in giving Shiatsu, the more relaxing is the effect. As you lean down, whether on to your palms or your thumbs, keep your arms and your shoulders relaxed. To help you, keep your arms very slightly bent – don't 'lock' them.

Make sure your pressure is perpendicular – if not, your partner may tilt forward or backward as you lean down on them. They should remain stable, and this is helped if you always support their back with the insides of your legs. When the pressure really penetrates, your partner will feel it down to the base of the spine.

Lifting and dropping the shoulders should be done again with the minimum of effort. Simply by bending and straightening your knees, and using your arms like a hook, you can raise your partner's arms and shoulders without using your muscles.

THE BENEFITS

Tension causes the shoulders literally to 'rise up'. This is quite visible in some people, who seem to carry their shoulders around their ears! By pushing down on them with natural, leaning pressure, you are assisting gravity to extend the muscles which have gradually contracted with tension. Using the thumbs, you can pay specific attention to the main offender – the trapezius muscle – and work at loosening it even further. The lift and drop works on the principle of first contracting then suddenly releasing the muscle, a kind of isometric exercise which relieves tightness and strengthens/tones the muscle.

Concentrate your thumb pressure on the gall bladder meridian, which runs along the top and back of the trapezius muscle. Imbalance in this meridian often leads to stiff shoulder muscles and joints. (Check the location of this meridian on pages 16–17.)

STEP 1 ▶

After finishing the final arm and shoulder stretch stand up behind your partner, supporting their back with the inside of your legs. Let them rest naturally against you. Place both your palms on their shoulders, letting your fingers fall over the tops of their arms. Keep your legs slightly bent and lean your body weight forward and down on to your palms, applying equal pressure simultaneously to the left and right and moving gradually out to the edge of the shoulders. Repeat several times.

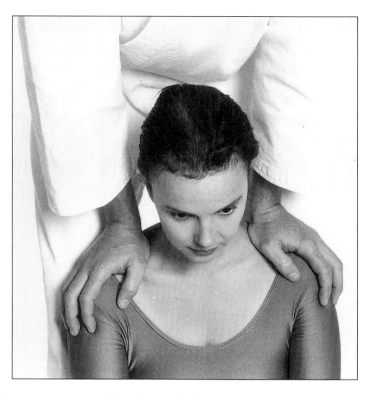

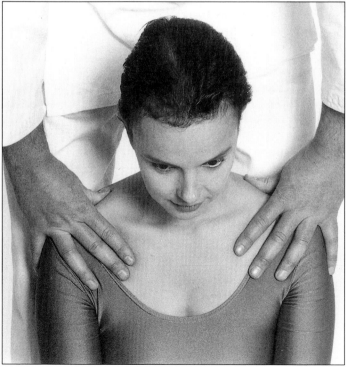

STEP 2 ◀

Keep your position, this time focusing your pressure on your thumbs instead of your palms. Allow your fingers to press gently against the top of your partner's chest, and with your thumbs trace horizontal lines on top of and around the back of the trapezius muscle. Maintain equal pressure both between left and right hands and between thumb and fingers of the same hand. Don't press too strongly with the thumbs, and distribute your body weight evenly, as these areas are often very sore! Hold each position for a few seconds, coordinate with your partner's breath and feel them relax into your pressure before moving on.

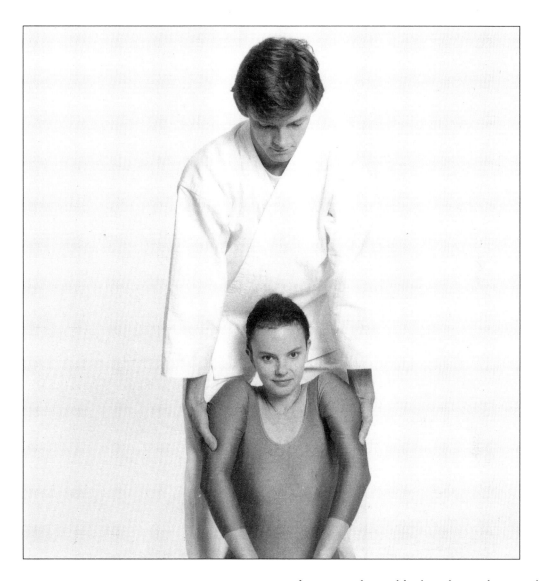

STEP 3 ▲

As you reach the outer edge of the shoulders, slide your palms over the tops of the arms and squeeze down both arms as far as the elbows, bending your knees as you go. In a semi-squatting position, holding your partner's arms at the elbows, straighten your legs and raise yourself upwards. Don't lift their arms, simply keep your own arms straight and relaxed and use them as 'hooks' so that as your body rises your arms follow, bringing their shoulders up with you. After holding the arms in the raised position for a few seconds, suddenly release them and let them drop to your partner's sides. Repeat several times. Ask your partner to breathe in with you as you raise their arms, and out as you drop them.

After completing the final lift and drop lean forward and squeeze down the arms again as far as the elbows. Turn your left foot sideways on to your partner's back supporting their spine all the way up with the side of your leg and prepare to give the upper body stretches ....

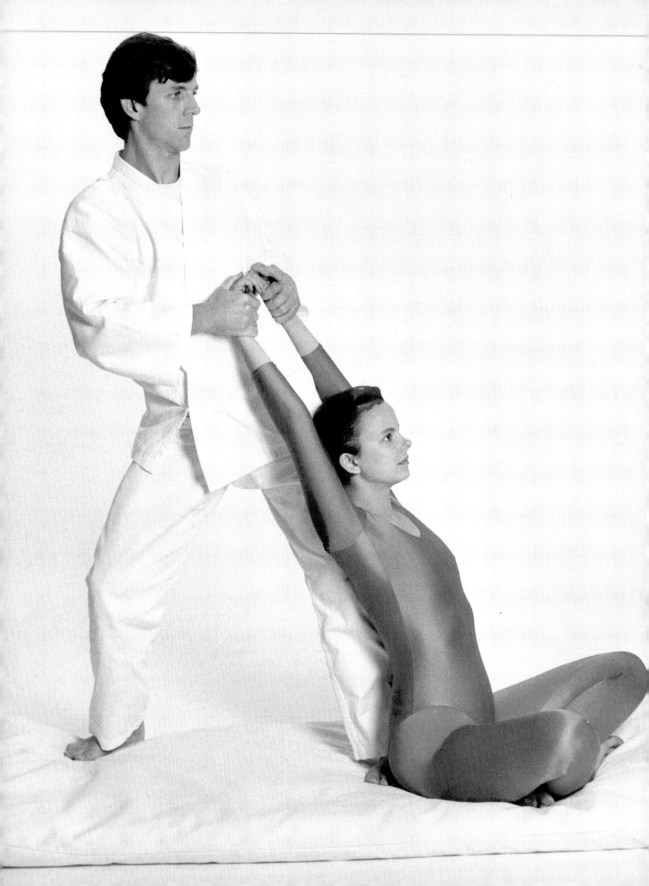

UPPER BODY STRETCH

This stretch is similar to the stretch given in the supine position (on page 141). In the sitting position, your partner's body has a much greater range of movement and the stretch can prove more effective.

However, because your partner doesn't have so much ground beneath them in this position you must provide all the necessary support throughout the whole movement. It is easy for them to tilt to the left or right and for you to lose your balance. If your partner feels unsteady they will tense their lower back muscles to keep themselves upright, and the full effect of the movement will be lost as they will resist the stretch.

Therefore body positioning is crucial. A sure way to know whether your positioning is right is to notice whether you have to make any undue effort in the movement. I have already stressed the importance of effortless movement in Shiatsu and this is especially relevant when giving stretches. If you rely on muscle power when stretching your partner's body, you will become tense, tire easily, and will always be limited by your own size and strength, and your partner's weight. With correct body positioning and appropriate timing even the smallest of people can stretch and manipulate the body with ease.

Once you have the mechanics sorted out, concentrate on the flow of the movement and the stretch will naturally become easier.

THE BENEFITS

This particular stretch is ideal for expanding the chest and opening up the shoulders, as well as for stretching the spine and arms. It rounds off the preparatory pressure, stretch and manipulative work we have already done to the whole upper body. It combines with them to offer the perfect solution to the stiffness and tightness of the neck, shoulders and back often caused by stress and poor posture (e.g. sitting hunched over a desk, VDU or steering wheel). When you feel you've got the weight of the world upon your shoulders or you feel constricted in the chest, this is the stretch for you!

In Shiatsu, we use this stretch to work principally on the Yin meridians of the arm, which include the heart, pericardium and lungs. It is especially effective for opening up the lungs, and you should ask your partner to breathe in deeply as you stretch open the chest and to breathe out as you relax the arms forward.

STEP 1 ▶

Having turned sideways after the shoulder pressure lift and drop, with the outside of your left leg supporting your partner's back, lean forward, sliding your hands down to your partner's wrists. At the same time, step back with your right foot, bending your knees and keeping your centre of gravity low. Don't allow your feet to be directly in line with one another, but keep them wide enough apart to give a solid base. Keep your partner stable by pressing the whole side of your leg against their spine, allowing them to relax against you.

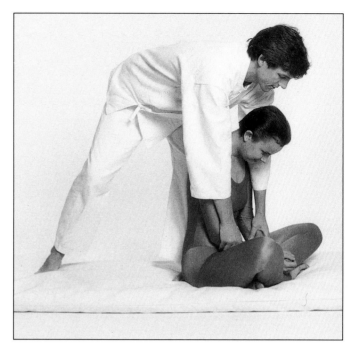

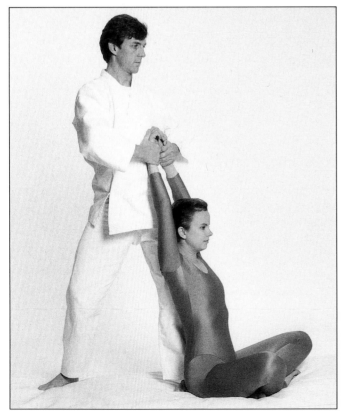

STEP 2 ◀

Lean forward and bring your partner's arms up in front of and above their head, still holding them gently but firmly by the wrists. Straighten your body and keep facing forward so that your partner's wrists come to rest against your chest, beginning to stretch their arms slightly.

STEP 3

Holding your partner's wrists firmly pressed against your chest and maintaining maximum contact up their back with the side of your left leg, begin

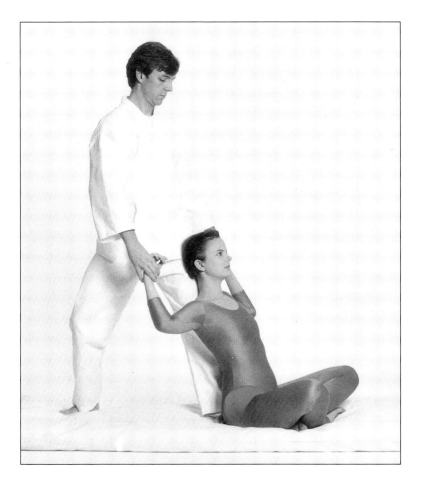

bending your right knee and leaning backwards directly away from your partner. Don't allow them to fall back beyond a 45° angle to the floor; otherwise you will have to lean too far backwards to achieve the stretch. So keep the outside of your left knee pressed into their back. Keep your upper body facing forward or your partner will tend to tilt to one side or the other. Keep your own spine straight by moving the hips instead of bending the upper body at the waist. Don't pull – simply lean back and the stretch will happen naturally without effort or strain (see the picture on page 48).

STEP 4 ▲

Ask your partner to breathe in during Step 3 and hold the stretch. As they breathe out, lean forward slightly, releasing them from the upward stretch but maintaining a chest-opening stretch as you guide their arms round and down to the original starting position. Repeat Steps 3 and 4 following the rhythm of your partner's breathing.

Note that you can step back with your left leg and support with your right during these steps if it is easier for you.

Finally, after finishing the last upper body stretch, release the arms completely, kneel behind your partner and 'wipe' down their spine with your palm, supporting their shoulder with your other hand. This completes the sitting position. Then ask them to lie on their front ready for the prone position . . . .

THE PRONE POSITION

Most people find this position very comfortable. However some e.g. those with heart or lung problems, or digestive or menstrual disorders, may experience discomfort caused by pressure on the chest or abdomen, and may only be able to lie in this position for a short time. A pillow under the chest may help, but it shouldn't be too soft or your partner will move about when you apply pressure.

Your partner will need to turn their head to one side. This may be difficult or uncomfortable for those with stiff or painful necks. If their neck is still stiff after the sitting position pressure, stretches and manipulations, go straight on to the supine position. In any case, remind your partner to turn their head to the opposite side from time to time to avoid stiffening up.

For the giver, this position is ideal for applying your full body weight by leaning over your partner and simply 'resting' on them. It is much easier to get a clear sense of the principles of Shiatsu in this position than, for example, in the sitting position where it is easy to use your muscle power instead.

Ideally, this position would follow on naturally from the sitting position, by which time your partner has had time to relax a little, you have loosened up their head, neck and shoulders and you will have 'tuned in' to their body, to assess their main areas of tension and weakness. Now they are ready to move into a more comfortable position and you are ready to begin a full body treatment.

THE BENEFITS

For the receiver, this position gives maximum attention to the back, an area with which many of us, through bad posture, injury or strain, may have some difficulty. Shiatsu to the whole back area never fails to bring relief to tired, aching or stiff muscles, relaxing the whole structure of the back. Minor self-adjustments in the spine often happen naturally during the treatment.

In oriental medicine the back, and more specifically points along the urinary bladder meridian which runs either side of the spine, are used a great deal in treatment. These points have particular significance in locating and treating imbalances in the whole body as they are related internally to all the major organs. Not unlike the branches of the central nervous system, they fan out from the spine to connect with the internal organs. Therefore treating the back may have a comprehensive effect on all the body systems.

ROCKING

After your partner has moved from the sitting position to lie down on their front, make sure their body is straight. You may need to stretch or move one of their legs or arms a little in order to do this as – when there is imbalance on one side of our body we often think we are positioned straight when we are in fact not.

Then, just to loosen them up in this position, and especially if you are beginning your treatment without any other preparatory work, just rock their body gently from side to side. Begin at the shoulders and, with your hands cupped, sway your body from side to side, alternately pushing and pulling their body with your cupped hands, moving gradually down towards the feet. You should create a kind of 'wave' effect which ripples through their body as you move. You can vary the strength and speed of this wave to suit your partner.

Note that for most of the prone position I am working on my partner's left side. This is usually more comfortable for right-handed people, though you can work from the other side if you find it more comfortable.

When your partner is fully relaxed in this position turn to face them sideways on, kneeling, ready to begin the back stretches ....

BACK STRETCHES

These are done as a preliminary warm-up to giving pressure on the back. I mentioned before that stretch work should always *follow* pressure. However in this case, it is not so much the muscles that are being stretched but the spine itself, and it feels good to have the back 'opened up' a little before receiving the focused pressure.

The main thing to concentrate on in giving these stretches is the correct positioning of your hands. This determines the direction of your pressure and hence the stretch. This time the direction is *not* perpendicular and you *do* maintain equal pressure on both hands.

There is no support hand and giving hand – both hands act as support and giving so that, in applying and releasing the pressure, you need to 'rock' back and forth gently (see pages 24–25).

Finally, these stretches are very subtle and *you* won't feel that much is happening. Check with your partner at first. Gradually you will get the 'feel' and be able to gauge it yourself.

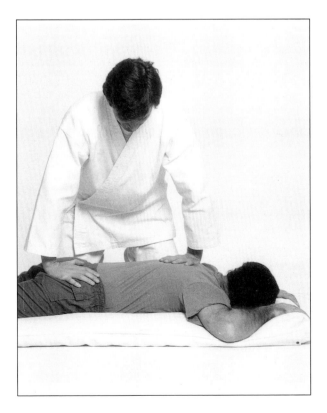

STEP 1 ◀

Kneel with your knees no wider than shoulder width apart, facing your partner with the centre of your body in line with the middle of their back. Lean forward and over your partner's back, extending your hands out in front of you to make contact. Your left hand should be on the near side shoulder blade, the right one on the far hip. Turn the fingers of both hands in to face each other and keep the arms slightly bent, elbows out. The action of leaning your body weight over and down, and the angle and positioning of your hands, should be enough to cause a stretch.

STEP 2

Release the stretch by rocking gently back into the upright position, releasing the pressure equally as you go. Change the position of the hands, moving the left one to the far shoulder blade, the right to the near side hip. Repeat the stretch as above in the opposite direction.

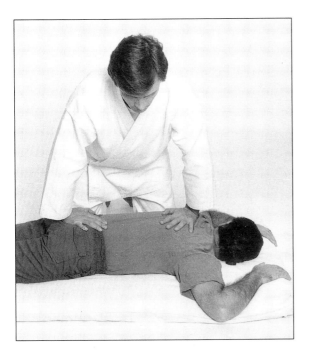

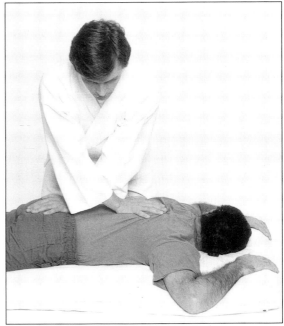

STEP 3 ▲

Release the stretch again and change the position of your hands, this time placing them centrally over the spine – the left hand at the upper end between the shoulder blades, the right at the lower end on the sacrum. Again, keep the fingers pointing inwards towards each other, arms bent, elbows out while you lean forward and over your partner to stretch the spine lengthways.

STEP 4 ▲

Release the stretch again by rocking back to the upright position, and cross your hands over in front of one another. Place them in the same positions as in Step 3, but this time with the left hand at the lower end of the spine and the right at the upper end. Now your fingers should be pointing away from each other but your arms should still be slightly bent, elbows out. Lean forward and over your partner to give a stretch lengthways to the spine – often a little stronger than the previous stretch.

STEP 5

In this position you can also stretch the muscles on either side of the spine. Adopt a similar position to that in Step 1, but place your left hand on the far shoulder blade (the same side as the right hand). With the fingers, arms and elbows in the same position, lean forward and over to give a stretch to the whole right (far) side of your partner's body. Change your hand positions to the near side and repeat the stretch to your partner's left side.

Release the final stretch and, keeping your position, lean forward and over your partner, extending both palms flat on to their back ready for 'palming' down the spine . . . .

PALMING DOWN THE SPINE

This is much like the palm pressure down the spine used in the 'First Contact' sequence in the sitting position (page 37). However, here you are able to apply more of your body weight when giving the pressure, as you are positioned above your partner, leaning over and down.

Don't 'bear down' on your partner by simply flopping your whole dead weight on to them; keep your chest open, head up and spine straight and just rest your weight on your partner. Keep your shoulders relaxed as you move, and always keep your arms slightly bent like a child's as it crawls. In fact this sequence is rather like learning to crawl again. Your arms are only used to support your body weight – you don't need to add any strength to the movement by pressing or pushing.

You can vary the amount of pressure applied by how far you lean over and also by the distance of your knees from your partner. The further from them you are, the more pressure will be applied when you lean over.

As in the sitting position, this palming movement tells you a lot about the state of the back, the location of weak or tense areas left and right, upper and lower. It is useful in giving pointers for more specific work later on.

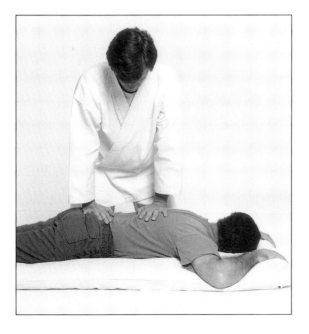

STEP 1 ◄

Having finished the spine stretches, lean forward and over your partner, keeping your same posture. Just when you are about to lose your balance and fall forwards, extend your palms to 'catch' yourself by placing them on your partner's back, side by side over the spine, fingers pointing away from you, applying equal pressure to each. Now begin shifting your weight smoothly from one palm to the other and 'walk' several times down the back, with the spine running under the centre of both your palms. Give equal pressure with the heel of your palms on the near side and your fingers on the far side.

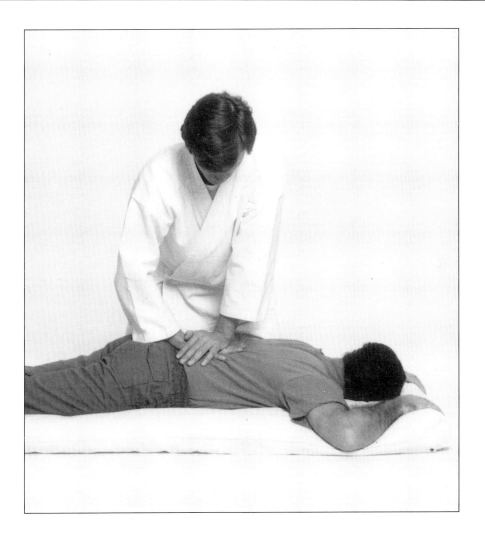

STEP 2 ▲

As you reach the base of your partner's spine for the last time, use your left palm to support your body weight and transfer your right palm back up to the top of the back, lengthways this time. Your fingers should be pointing up towards your partner's head, their spine running between your index and middle fingers. Take the weight on to your palm now and transfer your left hand up to the same position, placing your palm on top of and across your other hand, fingers pointing away from you. Now begin alternately applying and releasing your body weight on to your crossed palms as you gradually slide them down to the base of your partner's spine in a smooth, even movement. Repeat this several times.

As you reach the base of the spine for the last time, keep supporting your body weight with your right palm on your partner's sacrum and transfer your left hand to the upper back. Place your palm across the spine between the shoulder blades, fingers pointing away from you, and now transfer your weight on to this hand. Bend both arms and lean down to begin elbow Shiatsu to the mid-back : . . . .

MID-BACK

For practical reasons I have separated the back sequences into three parts, mid, upper and lower, each involving a different position.

For work on the mid-back I prefer using the elbows, which bring you closer to your partner and allow you a wider area of contact for pressure and support. When I say 'elbow' I actually mean a large area on the forearm below the elbow joint. The ball of the elbow itself is rarely, if ever, used, as it gives too strong pressure. I have also given an example of how to do the same sequences with your thumbs. But if you try this, make sure you keep your arms loose and don't tense your shoulders. The key to working with your elbow is to maintain good, firm support with the 'mother' hand (see principles of pressure in the chapter on the techniques of Shiatsu). In this way, because the elbow itself is less sensitive than your palm or fingers, you are feeling your way into the position using your support hand to gauge the amount of pressure and not simply leaning straight in with your elbow. In other words, the support hand takes *all* your weight at first, then gradually transfers some to the elbow until you reach equal pressure with both. You shift your position by taking the weight back on to the support hand and repeating the movement in a new location. This means there is *never* more weight on the elbow than on the support hand, and you can be sure to distribute your weight comfortably in this way.

THE BENEFITS

In any Shiatsu treatment it is vital to include work on the back; it relaxes and tones the muscles both structurally and energetically and thus restores a proper flow of energy to the meridians and the internal organs. For the most part you will be treating the two branches of the urinary bladder meridian (see pages 16–17), the first branch of which, running nearest the spine, has points with special connections to the internal organs (see benefits of the prone position on page 52). When treating the mid-back you can affect the digestive organs including the liver, gall bladder, spleen, pancreas and stomach. Thus as you follow this sequence we are having an effect on the urinary bladder channel itself, helping to relax the entire back which it governs, and also on the organs of digestion.

STEP 1

Having given crossed palm pressure down the spine for the last time, transfer your upper (left) palm to your partner's upper back and place it between their shoulder blades, fingers pointing away from you, with their spine running under the centre of your palm. Keep the same body position. Now shift your weight from your right to your left hand, removing the former from the lower back and bending the right arm at the elbow. With your right forearm parallel to the spine and about 2 inches (5 cm) from it on the far side (see the diagram on page 61) gently lower yourself on to your right elbow, gradually releasing and transferring pressure from support (left) to giving (right) arm until the pressure is equalised. Work down the mid-back in a smooth rhythm, transferring your body weight from support hand to giving elbow as you go, pausing to give equal pressure at each point for a few seconds. Repeat this line twice.

STEP 2 ▶

After giving elbow pressure to the first line twice, shift all your weight back on to your support (left) hand and lean a little further over your partner. Swivel your right arm at the shoulder so that your elbow turns outwards and your wrist inwards. Locate the second line (see diagram on page 61) and place your elbow below the shoulder blade. Momentarily shift your weight to your right elbow as you drop from your left palm on to your left elbow as support. Make sure you are relaxed in your new position before starting. Repeat this line twice.

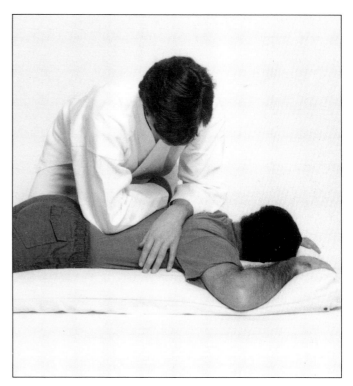

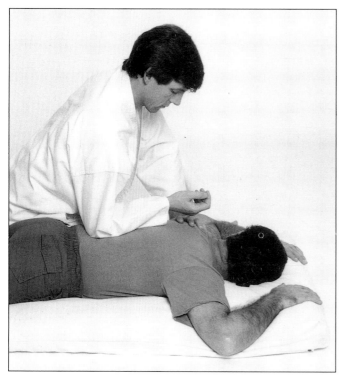

STEP 3 ◀

After giving elbow pressure to the second line twice on the far side of your partner, change to the near side. To do this, shift your weight from your support (left) forearm to your right hand, which you place on your partner's sacrum. Using your right hand as a pivot, swivel your body to face your partner's head and sit back on to your right heel, keeping your left knee up, foot flat on the floor. Now transfer your weight from right to left hand again, placing your left palm on the near shoulder blade. With this as your support, give elbow Shiatsu down the first line on the near side of your partner in the same smooth-flowing rhythm as before, elbow parallel to the spine.

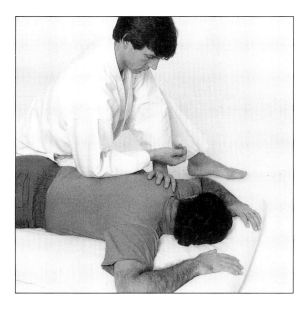

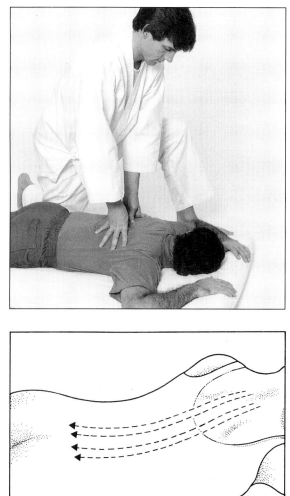

STEP 4 ▲

After giving elbow Shiatsu to the first line on your partner's near side twice, shift your weight on to your support (left) hand and swivel your right arm at the shoulder so your elbow turns outwards and your wrist inwards. Locate the second line (see the diagram to the right) and place your elbow, now at an angle to the spine, below their shoulder blade. Give Shiatsu down this line from top to bottom, alternately shifting your weight on to support and giving arms.

Position if using thumbs ▲ ▶

If you prefer to use your thumbs instead of your elbows follow the same two lines on either side of your partner from top to bottom of the back. Your position must change: kneeling up on your right knee, the left foot flat on the floor. In this position you can lean over and down on to your partner, using both hands on either side of the spine simultaneously. Thus you can give thumb Shiatsu to both first lines and both second lines in the same movement. For this movement you will have to 'rock' in and out and not tense your arms and shoulders.

Pressure lines ▲

These are the lines to follow when applying your pressure. The first, about 2 inches (5 cm) either side of the spine, is located in a natural channel or valley which runs parallel to the spine in between two muscles. It is relatively easy to locate. The second line is the same distance again from the spine as the first, but a little more difficult to locate. Angle your forearm to give pressure to the second line so that it slots comfortably into the spaces between the ribs.

SHOULDERS, UPPER BACK AND ARMS

Now you can return to work on an area you have already loosened up in the sitting position. This time you will be able to work on top of, as well as around, the shoulder blade and give Shiatsu to both sides of the arms. You will also be able to reach the upper back, between the shoulder blades.

This sequence involves a major change of position, with you kneeling above your partner's head. Make sure you are comfortable – use a cushion if you need one, or make sure you are kneeling on the futon or mattress. Try to be as smooth as possible in the moving from one position to the next, in order not to interrupt the flow of your treatment. As always, don't at any time break contact with your partner.

The main things to be aware of here are angle of pressure and weight distribution. To give pressure to the upper back you will need to be kneeling up so that your weight is properly over your partner. To give pressure around the tops of the shoulder blades you will need to keep your hips low so that you can lean forward rather than down. Because of the curve of the upper back, there will be various positions between these two extremes and you will have to adjust your body weight accordingly to keep the pressure perpendicular. Similarly, be careful to distribute your weight evenly, especially when 'walking' down the arms with your palms, since excessive pressure on the shoulder joint can be painful.

THE BENEFITS

As mentioned in the sitting position shoulder sequences (page 45), many people suffer from stiffness and pain in these areas and Shiatsu is especially effective at relieving it. The added benefits of working in this position are that you are able to use more of your body weight in the movements and to sustain the pressure for longer, as both you and your partner are more stable and comfortable in the prone position.

In Shiatsu you can work, as mentioned, along and behind the trapezius muscle and either side of the spine, concentrating on the urinary bladder, gall bladder and small intestine meridians – the most common site of blockage of vital energy, causing stiffness and pain in these areas. The upper back, between the shoulder blades, is associated with heart and lung function in oriental medicine, and you can affect these organs by work in this area following both the urinary bladder lines (see the diagrams on pages 16–17).

STEP 1

After finishing elbow Shiatsu to the second bladder line on your near side, swing up to kneel at your partner's head, facing down towards their feet. Use your right arm as a pivot to take your body weight as you swing around, and try to make the movement as smooth as possible. Once you are kneeling above your partner, with their head between your knees, lean forward, extend your arms in front of you and make contact with your palms on your partner's shoulders. 'Tune in' to your partner in this new position and notice any particular tensions under your palms.

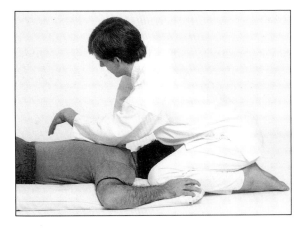

STEP 2 ◀

After giving equal pressure to your partner's shoulders (Step 1), transfer all your weight to one hand and begin to work around the inside edge of the shoulder blade with your elbow. As usual, release your weight gradually from the support hand to the giving elbow until equal pressure is achieved. Hold the pressure a few seconds before moving on to the next point. Keep your shoulders loose and use the edge of your forearm. Repeat the movement to the other side. Give pressure to the less tense side first.

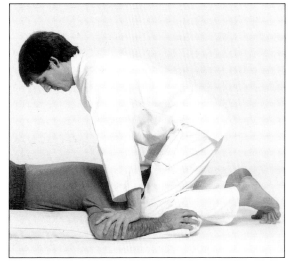

STEP 3 ◀

After giving elbow pressure around the top of both shoulder blades, kneel up, placing both palms on top of the shoulders and applying equal pressure. Begin to 'walk' your palms down your partner's arms by alternately releasing and applying pressure with each palm in turn. Gradually work your way down to the hands, holding equal pressure on both hands with your palms to finish. Repeat the movement. As you 'walk' down your partner's arms, allow your hips to sink back naturally towards the floor, keeping your body weight directly over your palms at all times.

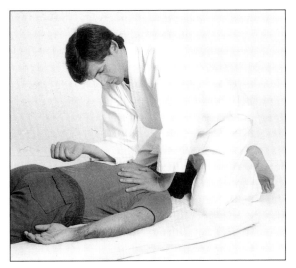

STEP 4 ◀

As you reach your partner's hands for the second time, tuck their arms under and down by their sides one by one. With their arms in this new position it is easier to give elbow pressure to the two bladder lines (see the diagram on page 61). Kneel up and, supporting yourself with one palm on your partner's shoulder, give elbow Shiatsu to the two bladder lines on the other side of their back. Begin roughly at the point you began to work down the back in the mid-back sequences on page 59, this time working up the back towards yourself. Sink your hips as you go in order to keep your pressure perpendicular. Repeat the movement on the other side. As above, begin with the less tense side first.

STEP 5

As you finish giving elbow pressure to the bladder lines on your partner's second side, return to the first side using the same support on the shoulder and preparing to work with the elbow in the same way as in Step 2. But this time give elbow Shiatsu widthways across the shoulder blade itself, on the bone. Lean your body weight sideways as you go, finishing up with your elbow in the soft flesh at the back of your partner's armpit. Repeat on the other side.

STEP 6

After giving pressure to the second shoulder blade, kneel up, placing both palms on your partner's shoulders and applying equal pressure with your palms. In the same way as Step 3, begin 'walking' down your partner's arms. This time, however, move your body weight forward rather than back, once again ending up by giving alternate palm pressure as far as your partner's palms.

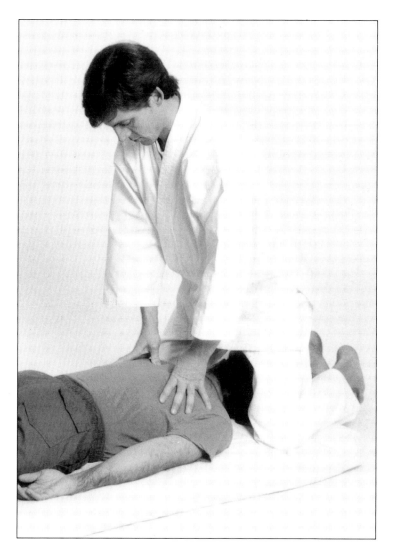

Position if using thumbs ◄
Steps 2–6 can also be done with your thumbs instead of your elbows. Pay attention to proper support and positioning and don't tense your arms and shoulders. Follow all the sequences in terms of your body positioning, simply substituting your thumbs and fingers for your elbows. The only difference is that you will work on both shoulders/bladder lines/shoulder blades at the same time, rather than one by one.

After 'walking' down your partner's arms for the last time lean forward and over their back, placing both your palms either side of their spine, and get ready to give palm pressure down the back . . . .

PALMING DOWN THE BACK

Now that you have given pressure to both the mid- and upper back, you are in an ideal position to lean over your partner and palm down their whole back on both sides. The advantage of being above their head rather than to one side of them is that it is easier to give equal pressure on both palms, as the centre of their back is directly under the centre of your chest.

Your palms should be either side of the spine, heels of the palms facing each other, with the fingers pointing outwards across the side of their body. Make sure you don't place any direct pressure on the spine – the heels of your palms should be far enough apart that the spine runs in the gap between them. Keep maximum contact between the surface of your palms and your partner's back.

There are two possible movements in this sequence, either using both palms at the same time, with equal pressure, or shifting the weight alternately on to each palm one by one like a 'walk'. Double-handed pressure will mean you must 'rock' in and out of position to apply the pressure, whilst alternate-handed pressure will allow you to maintain constant pressure throughout, shifting the weight back and forth to each hand in turn. Either method or both is fine.

As usual with this type of palm pressure, pay attention to not tensing your shoulders and arms and get a nice rhythm going as you move down the spine.

THE BENEFITS

This is really a finishing-off sequence to the pressure you have already been giving to the back. It smooths over the areas you have worked on in detail and concludes the movement with a nice spine stretch, which gives your partner's back a final loosening up before you move on.

It is also a chance for you to check your work and see how effective it has been in releasing any tension that you may have felt in certain areas earlier on.

The overall effect of this sequence can be compared to the most basic stroke in massage, 'effleurage', because of its smooth, rhythmic flow and general relaxing effect.

STEP 1

After 'walking' down your partner's arms to their palms for the last time, rock back and then up on to your knees again, placing your palms one on either side of their spine at the top of their back. The heels of your palms should be facing each other and your partner's spine running in between, with your fingers pointing away across the sides of their back. Now give palm pressure to both sides of their back from top to bottom, with both hands at once or with each hand alternately. You will need to 'rock' your body forward and back to apply double-handed pressure while you simply 'walk' your palms down the back to apply alternate pressure with each hand in turn, maintaining constant pressure as you go. Repeat the sequence several times.

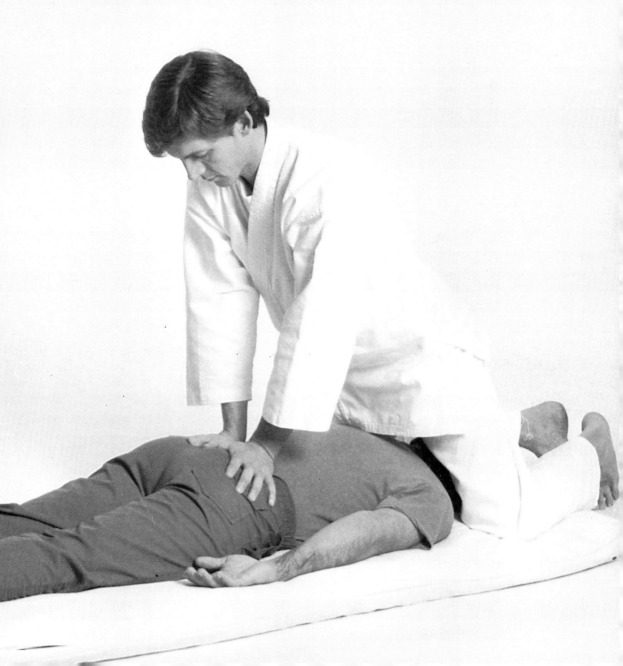

STEP 2 ▼

After finishing palm pressure down the back, rock back upright and sink into the kneeling position, resting on the backs of your heels. Place your palms on top of one another over your partner's spine at the top of their back. Keeping your hips low, lean forward and allow your body weight to slide your hands along the spine at the bottom. At the point of your maximum extension the heel of your palms will usually catch the base of your partner's spine and hold you there, preventing you from going any further. It is this which allows the spine stretch to happen. Remember to keep your hips near the floor and give almost horizontal pressure along the spine. If you rise up on to your knees and press downwards you will never achieve the stretch.

After finishing the spine stretch lean back, place your left palm on the floor under your partner's right armpit and swivel round to your partner's side, using your arm as a pivot. Position yourself at your partner's side, kneeling to face them at the level of their lower back, ready to begin Shiatsu to this area . . . .

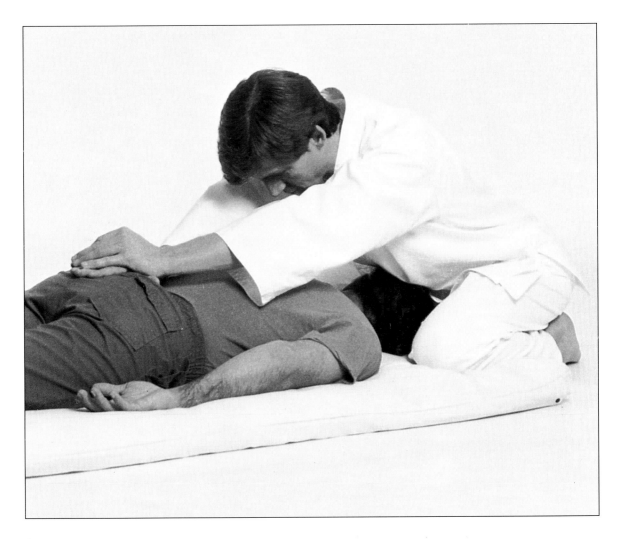

LOWER BACK

Having completed the mid- and upper back work, you can now focus on the last section, the lower part. Whilst the other two areas were fairly firm, well-muscled and in places bony, this area is essentially soft, in between the ribs and the pelvis. Because there is no bony protection, and because the kidneys are here, take care not to give any sudden, strong pressure with any sharp part of your anatomy. Don't, for example, use the ball of your elbow, but rather your forearm below the elbow joint.

Because this can be a delicate area to work in, your support must be especially firm. So pick the largest, fleshiest area to support your body weight – the buttocks. However, the buttocks can often be tender themselves, so don't dig your support elbow in suddenly or too deeply!

To apply pressure to this area, kneel alongside your partner, facing them at the level of the lower back, having moved back round from above their head. This involves quite a big movement which needs to be performed quickly but without effort or strain, maintaining contact with your partner at all times and where possible keeping a sense of flow in the sequence.

THE BENEFITS

For some people, the lower back can be a weak spot. Whenever we are under extra strain there is often one particular area which repeatedly gives us problems, and it may well be the lower back. Receiving Shiatsu pressure in this area usually feels comforting and can begin to release tension and strain as well as restore a proper flow of energy, invigorating and stimulating it.

In oriental medicine the lower back is associated with the kidney and urinary bladder, and in treating this area we can affect these organs and help balance the flow of energy in their respective meridians. Imbalance in these two organ and meridian systems is often seen as the primary cause of much lower backache. We can also hope to affect the functioning of the intestines, particularly the lower intestines, with pressure in this area.

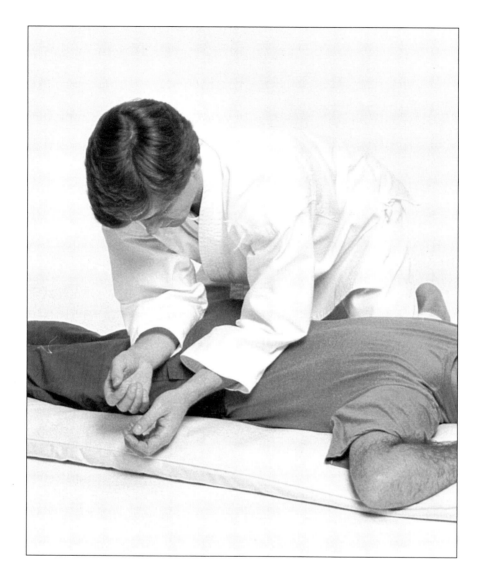

STEP 1 ▲

After swivelling round from above your partner's head, using your left arm as a pivot, kneel to face them at the level of their lower back. Kneel up and lean forward and over them, extending your right forearm and placing it on the fleshiest part of their far (right) buttock. Now place your left forearm across the far side of their lower back and gradually transfer your weight from the right to the left arm until you have equalised the pressure. Gradually work your way along a horizontal line in the small of the back from near the spine over to the side of the body. The further over you go, the more you will need to kneel up and lean over and the firmer your support will need to be.

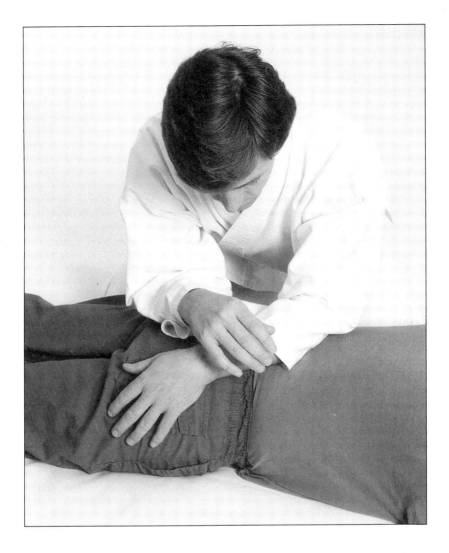

STEP 2 ▲

After finishing pressure to the far side of your partner's lower back sit back on to your heels, releasing your pressure and sliding both elbows to your partner's near side. Place them in the same positions as in Step 1, support your elbow on their buttock and give elbow Shiatsu in the soft part of the lower back near the spine. Keeping your hips low and without kneeling up, lean forward, taking your weight on to your support elbow. Transfer your weight to the giving (left) elbow and equalise the pressure. Gradually work along a similar horizontal line as in Step 1, from nearest the spine to the side of your partner's body. Make sure you are kneeling far enough from your partner not to get cramped during this movement. Maintain the angle of your pressure perpendicular at all times by keeping your hips low.

After finishing pressure to the near side lower back, turn to face your partner's head, kneeling up on the right knee and stepping forward with the left foot, ready to begin thumb pressure to the sacrum . . . .

SACRUM

In Shiatsu we use various parts of our body to apply pressure, and each is used for a different reason and effect (see page 27). The thumbs are especially useful for working on small, detailed areas such as the face and neck, the feet and hands, and, in this case, the sacrum. The sacrum is a triangular-shaped bone at the base of the spine which runs from the top of the pelvis down to the tip of the coccyx (tail bone). Since it is an integral part of the spine, the back sequence would be incomplete without working on it.

Give equal pressure with both hands while distributing your weight equally over the thumb and fingers of each hand – don't focus your pressure too much on the thumbs alone.

After a few treatments on different people you will get used to the shape of the sacrum and your thumbs will naturally find their way along the lines (see diagram opposite). As a guide, try to find the small depressions either side of the centre of the sacrum which run along the first line.

THE BENEFITS

The sacral area is used a lot in Shiatsu to treat a variety of aches, pains and other symptoms of external and internal origin. Lower backache, sciatica, leg and buttock tension and pain can all be helped from this area. These symptoms may be caused by structural imbalance, which Shiatsu can help to correct – however, pains in this area often have an internal origin and may be linked to menstrual or uro-genital disorders. Therefore this is one of the areas used to help regulate such problems as painful or irregular menstruation, frequent urination, urine retention and impotence. Once again the urinary bladder channel runs over this area – hence the effect on that meridian and organ system.

STEP 1 ▶

Turn to face your partner's head from the kneeling position, keeping your right knee on the floor and stepping up with the left foot. Place both hands on your partner's sacral area with your thumbs either side of the centre of the sacrum and your fingers spread out over the buttocks. Lean forward and slightly to the side so that your weight is directly over your hands and begin applying equal pressure on to both hands, spreading the weight evenly over your fingers and thumbs.

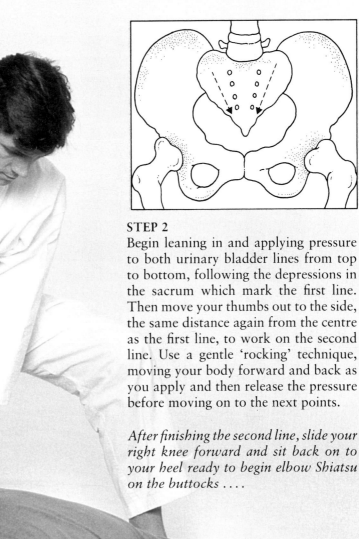

STEP 2

Begin leaning in and applying pressure to both urinary bladder lines from top to bottom, following the depressions in the sacrum which mark the first line. Then move your thumbs out to the side, the same distance again from the centre as the first line, to work on the second line. Use a gentle 'rocking' technique, moving your body forward and back as you apply and then release the pressure before moving on to the next points.

After finishing the second line, slide your right knee forward and sit back on to your heel ready to begin elbow Shiatsu on the buttocks ....

BUTTOCKS

Since the buttocks are large and fleshy you can work on them with your elbows to great effect. The region you want to reach includes all the muscle either side of the sacrum round as far as the hipbone. Since this is a large, rounded area you need to adopt different positions to maintain perpendicular pressure.

The most obvious place for your support hand is the lower back, but make sure that part of your palm is placed on the upper part of the sacral area rather than the small of the back, which is naturally less strong.

By adopting two different positions relative to your partner, rather like you did for the mid-back sequence (page 60), you can reach both sides of your partner's buttocks without crossing over them.

As these areas often carry a lot of tension, especially in men, make sure that your pressure is applied slowly, evenly and without pushing. Don't make any sudden movements, and lower yourself gently into position by transferring weight from the support elbow to the giving elbow. Don't lean heavily straight on to the giving elbow!

THE BENEFITS

The buttocks often carry a great deal of tension, which may be referred from the back as a result of lumbago caused by bad posture, injury or chronic distortion of the spine. Equally, internal imbalances such as constipation, irregular menstruation or uro-genital problems can cause tightness and pain in this area. Such tension can be eased with Shiatsu, which in turn helps regulate deeper, internal imbalances. The urinary bladder and gall bladder meridians are the main ones to focus on here, the urinary bladder for such problems as mentioned in the sacrum sequence (see page 72) and the gall bladder for tension and tightness in the buttocks, hips and legs. Of particular use is the gall bladder point in the centre of the buttock (in the natural depression when the buttocks are tensed), which is very effective in treating sciatic pain.

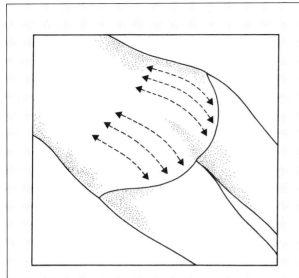

STEP 1

After finishing pressure to the second bladder line on the sacrum, slide the right knee forward and sit back on your right heel, your hips roughly level with your partner's. Lean to your right, over your partner, placing your left palm over their sacrum in the middle and taking your weight on to it. Now bring your right elbow over to the right buttock area and begin working near the centre crease of the buttocks, from just below the underside of the sacrum down to the upper thigh.

Follow three vertical lines from top to bottom of the buttock (see diagram), shifting your pressure further over your partner for each line in order to maintain equal pressure. Use your left foot as a counter-weight to your upper body by extending it out to the side the further you lean over to the right. Repeat each line twice.

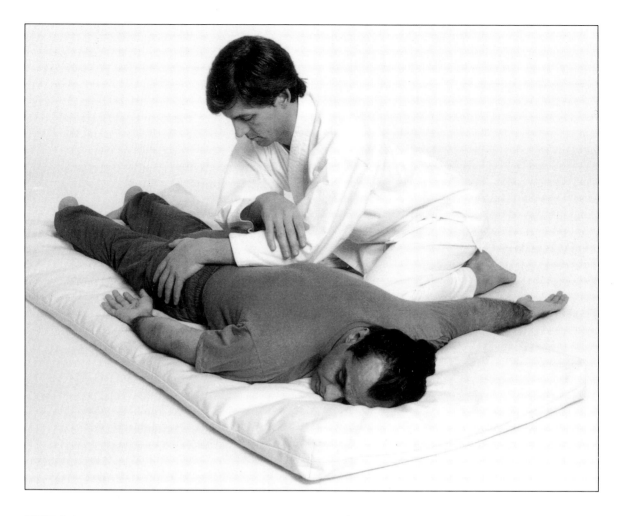

STEP 2 ▲

After finishing pressure to the far (right) buttock, swivel back to face your partner, kneeling, level with their hips. Lean forward, placing your left forearm over the sacral area for support and leaning your body weight over and down on to it. Don't bear your weight down on them – simply rest gently against them.

Place your right forearm lengthways on the first of the three buttock lines (see diagram on page 75), starting at the top under the sacrum. Shift your weight from support elbow to giving elbow until it equalises, and in this way work down the three lines in turn, gradually sinking your hips as you go on to maintain perpendicular pressure.

The three lines on the buttocks run parallel with each other from just below the underside of the edge of the sacrum down to the top of the thigh. The first lies close to the centre of the buttock crease, about the same distance from it as the first urinary bladder line in the sacrum sequence (see page 73). The second two lines are equal distances apart, spanning the entire width and length of the buttock area as far across as the hip joint and the side of the hip. In following the three lines, you should cover the whole buttock area.

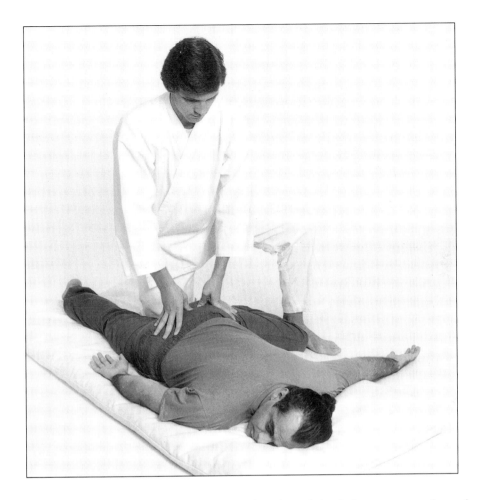

STEP 3 ▲

If you want to focus specifically on the buttock area because it is particularly tight or in need of attention, use your thumbs instead of or as well as your elbows. Take hold of your partner's left foot with your right hand, and guiding their leg with your left hand, slide it up along the floor at right-angles so their knee comes up level with their hip. Kneeling with your right knee between their legs, your left foot on the floor outside their left knee lean over and down, placing your palms on their left buttock, your thumbs together, fingers pointing out to the sides. Give two-handed Shiatsu to all three lines on the buttocks (see the diagram on page 75) from the inside out, 'rocking' your body weight back and forth as you go. Give equal pressure with both

hands and don't focus too much on the thumbs, spreading your weight evenly over your whole hand. Return the left leg to the straight position, cross over your partner to their right side and repeat the sequence to their right leg.

After finishing thumb or elbow Shiatsu to the buttocks, shift your body position down towards your partner's feet slightly, bringing the centre of your body in line with their thigh. Place your left palm on their sacrum for support, pick up their right lower leg at the ankle and prepare to begin knee Shiatsu to the thigh . . . .

LEGS

When working with the arms and legs, you can adjust the position of your partner's limb to suit your angle of pressure without having to alter your own position dramatically. This is because the ball and socket joint (in the hip and in the shoulder) allows a very wide and varied angle of movement. This is useful, as it allows you to maintain a very stable, relaxed position throughout the movements, getting your partner's limb to 'do the work' for you.

Your positioning is important, as you must not over-reach in order to give pressure as far as the feet. If your partner has long legs it may be necessary to shift your position down towards the feet and palm down the legs in two separate movements. The main rule is not to spread your palms wider than shoulder width apart when working down the legs, as this will unbalance you.

Generally the backs of the legs are strong, well-muscled areas and you can give Shiatsu effectively to a wide area using the knee. However, the backs of the calves can often be tender and here it is advisable to use elbow or palm pressure. One area that is especially tender and can be considered a 'weak spot' is the back of the knee. Never give full pressure to this area, and when working over it simply pass lightly over the top, maintaining contact but applying no pressure.

The most comfortable position for your partner is with their legs close together, toes turned in, heels flopping out. Some people with particularly stiff ankles and toes may not be able to maintain this position and their heels will flop inwards with their toes pointing out. Be careful with the angle of your pressure when palming down these people's lower legs.

THE BENEFITS

The extremities (arms and legs) often suffer as a result of an internal balance in the centre of the body: for example, circulatory problems of the heart will invariably lead to coldness of the limbs and may include accumulation of fluids (oedema). Constipation usually causes a heavy, dull sensation in the legs, whilst a low back injury may cause pain down one or both sides of the legs.

Shiatsu treatment of the legs is very important in restoring the proper flow of energy, blood and body fluids in the local area as well as to the rest of the body. Cramps, chills, fluid retention, numbness, pain and injury to the soft tissues (muscles, ligaments and tendons) can all be treated from the legs.

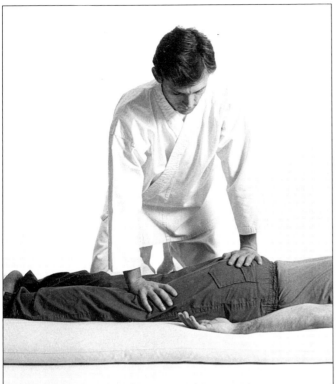

After completing work on the buttocks, shift your position down towards your partner's feet, bringing the centre of your body in line with their thigh. Before beginning knee pressure, however, palm down the far (right) and near (left) leg from under the buttocks to the feet. Remember to release pressure as you pass over the back of the knee, and to shift your body position down towards your partner's feet to avoid over-reaching yourself.

STEP 1 ▶

Place your left hand on the sacrum to support your body weight. Pick up the near (left) lower leg at the ankle with your right hand, and bring it towards you to rest against your right hip. Take your weight equally on to your left knee and left hand and raise your right knee, placing it gently in position on the back of your partner's thigh below the left buttock. Don't apply pressure immediately; get comfortable in this position first and then gradually, as always, transfer your body weight from your left knee and palm on to your right knee until all three points receive equal pressure. Don't hang back with your hips. Lean over fully, but make sure you don't bear your weight down on your partner. Gradually work down the thigh as far as the knee. Repeat this line twice.

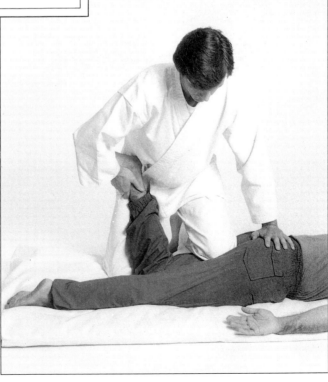

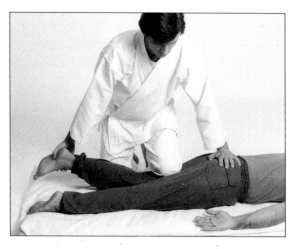

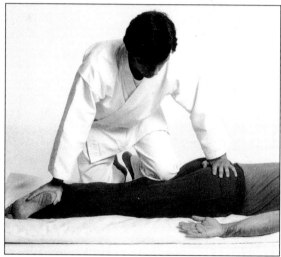

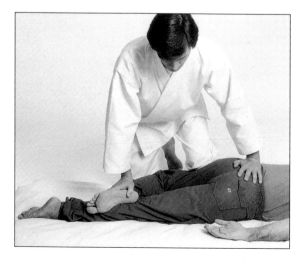

STEP 2 ◄

Lower your partner's leg until it almost touches the floor, holding it by the ankle with your cupped right palm. Keep your support hand (left) on the sacrum. Repeat twice the same knee sequence as in Step 1.

STEP 3 ▼ ◄

Fold your partner's left ankle over the back of their right heel, placing your right palm over the top to take your weight. Keep your support hand on the sacrum and lean forward to take your weight equally on both palms. Simultaneously bring your left knee up to make thigh contact just under the buttock. When properly balanced and supported, give knee Shiatsu along a line midway between the back and the side of the thigh as far as the knee. Repeat twice. Continue the line down the lower leg by changing knees, placing your left knee on the floor and raising the right to continue giving pressure without moving the support hands. Repeat this line twice.

STEP 4 ▼ ◄

Now take hold of your partner's left ankle and lean back, holding the ankle to chest and sliding their left knee out to the side. Lean forward again, folding the ankle over the back of their calf so the leg forms a V. Lean your body weight forward, supporting it equally on both hands, and place your left knee in position on the side of your partner's leg just below the hip joint. Give knee Shiatsu along a line which runs along the side of the leg as far as their knee. Repeat this line twice. Then, as in Step 3, continue down the lower leg by changing knees. Repeat twice.

Lean back, bringing your partner's ankle to your chest and guiding their knee back to its original position with your left hand so that the leg is straight again. Slide your right knee forward, allowing their lower leg to rest on top of it, and prepare to give elbow Shiatsu to the calf. . . .

CALVES, ANKLES AND FEET

In the previous sequences the ball and socket joint of the hip allowed you to rotate your partner's thigh into the desired position. But here you must alter your own position in order to reach the necessary areas for treatment.

If you are fairly flexible, adopt a wide-knee posture with one knee up on the back of your partner's thigh (see picture on next page). But if it is difficult for you to stretch that knee up on to the thigh, keep it on the ground. Just make sure you are comfortable.

Many people experience tenderness and pain in the calf muscles and meridians, so be careful with the pressure you apply and give proper support. Again, keep clear of the tender back of the knee when giving elbow pressure. When working in the calf area you may use both elbows, or you may support your body weight by placing one palm on the sole of your partner's foot and working along the calf with one elbow. Make sure your pressure is perpendicular and equal.

When working on the ankles and feet, use your elbows or thumbs or both. As these are important areas you will return to them later in the supine position sequences.

THE BENEFITS

The further from the centre of the body you go, the more severe may be the effect of any circulatory and neurological problems. Shiatsu to the calves and feet can restore proper energy flow and help improve circulation of blood and body fluids to these areas and to the body as a whole. This will help problems such as cold feet, water retention in the ankles and feet, muscle cramps, sciatica, numbness and pain, as well as improve mobility and reduce stiffness and swelling due to injury.

All the meridians run to the feet and toes, but in addition there are special reflex areas on the soles which, when stimulated, are considered to have a regulating effect on the internal organ systems as a whole.

In oriental medicine flexibility of the ankles, feet and toes (as well as wrists, hands and fingers) is considered very important to one's general state of health. This reflects the fact that the energy circulating in the meridians crosses from one meridian network to the next in these areas, so that any blockages here will have a knock-on effect on the entire system.

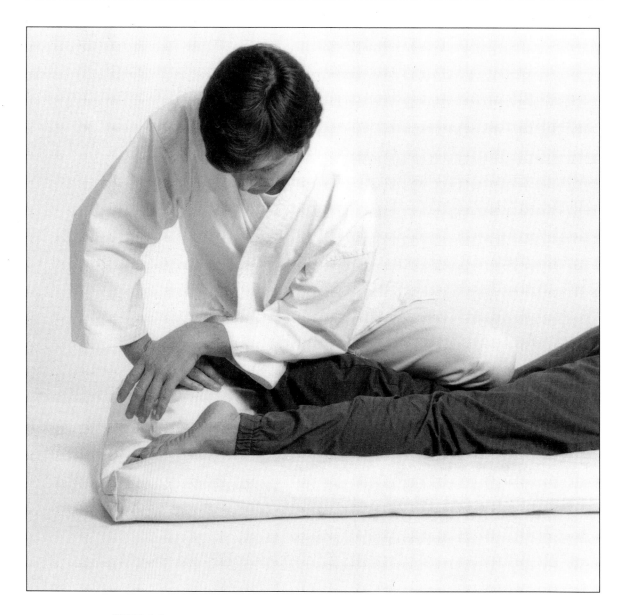

STEP 1 ▲

After finishing knee Shiatsu to the last line down the side of your partner's leg, return the leg to the straight position, sliding your right knee forward and allowing their ankle to rest on top of it. Lift your left knee up on top of the back of your partner's thigh (or leave it on the ground if more comfortable) and lean forward placing your right palm on the sole of your partner's foot for support. Then use your left elbow to give Shiatsu along the calf.

STEP 2 ▶

After finishing elbow Shiatsu along the calf, place your right palm on the upturned sole of your partner's left foot for support. Lean forward and place your left elbow on the Achilles tendon. Equalise your pressure and gently rotate the ankle back and forth with your right hand, so that your elbow pressure is applied to the top and sides of the Achilles tendon in turn.

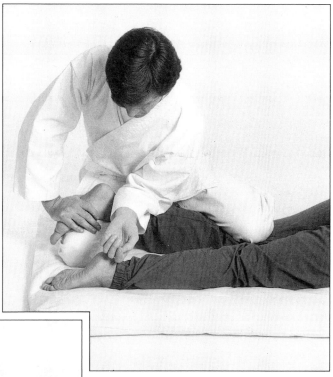

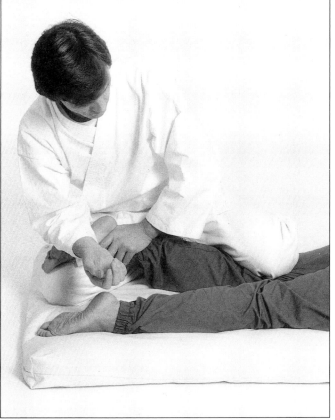

STEP 3 ◀

Maintain your body position but swap hand positions, placing your left palm over the back of your partner's ankle and supporting your body weight on it. Drop your right forearm down to rest on the sole of their foot, then transfer the weight over from support arm to giving arm until you reach equal pressure. Give pressure across the sole of the foot from the heel to back of the toes. Make sure your right knee is directly under your partner's foot, supporting it fully. You may need to slide it further down following the previous sequence.

After giving pressure to the sole of the foot, pick up your partner's leg at the ankle, turning to face up towards their head and kneeling to secure their knee between both your knees, ready to shake and rotate the ankle . . . .

ROTATIONS AND STRETCHES
(Feet, Ankles and Legs)

Once again, following pressure which loosens an area up, freeing blocked energy and balancing the flow, you can stretch and manipulate the area to enhance the overall effect. Now you can further loosen the ankle and toe joints as well as giving a good stretch to the whole leg. These movements complete the work on your partner's left leg. Then you will change sides and repeat the whole series of sequences from 'Legs' (page 78), to finish with these same stretches and manipulations before moving on to work on both legs at the same time.

The ankles can often become stiff and will resist passive movement. Just as people may try to assist you in moving their neck when you don't want them to, so they may find it hard simply to relax their ankles and let you do the rotations. Don't force the movement. The most effective remedy for an 'over-helpful' ankle is a firm but relaxed shake. And don't focus too hard on the movement or rotate too slowly and deliberately. Keep the movement soft but free and open, making nice, big, loose circles. The more relaxed you are, the more they will sense this and relax themselves.

THE BENEFITS

A great deal of stagnation of energy, blood and fluid circulation occurs in the legs through lack of adequate movement and exercise in the lower body. The orientals have the advantage of sitting habits which maintain a great deal of flexibility and strength in the legs and particularly in the ankles, feet and toes. In the West, however, a more sedentary lifestyle and a less demanding sitting posture have contributed to stiffness and inflexibility in the knee, ankle and toe joints, which gets worse through lack of movement and exercise. These sequences are a passive form of exercise which return a measure of flexibility to these key areas and restore balance to the whole lower body.

In oriental medicine it is said that energy and blood flow abundantly through the joints, so that to keep them soft and supple has preventive implications for problems such as arthritis, gout, varicose veins, oedema, poor circulation, cramps, numbness and pain.

STEP 1 ▶

After finishing elbow and thumb pressure to the sole of the foot, pick up your partner's left leg at the ankle with your right hand and swivel round to face their head, securing their knee between both your knees and kneeling back on to your heels.

Taking hold of their left ankle in both hands, shake it gently but firmly back and forth to loosen it up. Use your whole body weight in the movement, not just your arms or hands.

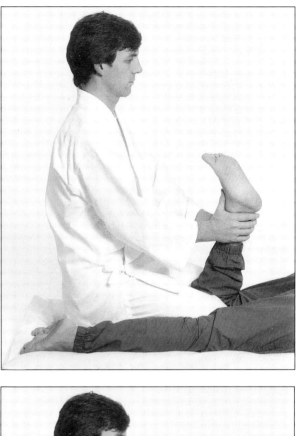

STEP 2 ▶

Keeping your left hand in place firmly grasping the outside of their ankle, use your right hand to begin giving ankle rotations in both directions. Keep their leg steady with your supporting hand. Don't allow it to wave around – only the foot should move. Make nice, big, loose movements, stopping to shake and loosen your partner's ankle if you feel it stiffening up during the rotation.

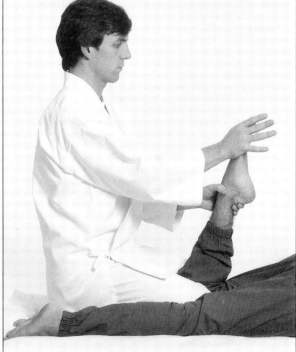

STEP 3 ▶

After rotating the ankle in both directions, kneel up and, keeping your right knee on the ground, step out with the left foot about level with your partner's hip. Keep holding their ankle firmly in your left hand and place your right palm on top of the upturned sole of their foot, laying it flat across it. Lean your body weight down on to the sole of the foot, gradually stretching the back of the Achilles tendon. Then lean forward, keeping the foot stretch on, guiding your partner's heel towards the centre of their left buttock. Move your whole body with their foot – don't just use your palm to give the stretch. Try to judge the maximum comfortable extent of the stretch for your partner without having to wait for some sort of reaction.

Alternatively, or in addition, you can use your forearm instead of your palm.

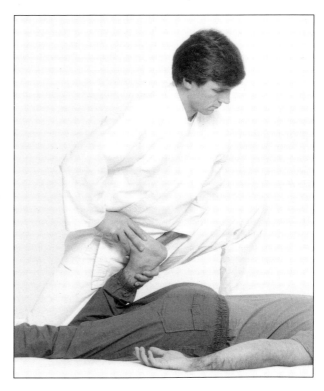

STEP 4 ▶

After holding the Achilles stretch for a few seconds, lean back a little and momentarily release your elbow or palm from the sole of your partner's foot. Catch the top of their toes with your right palm and fold them up and away from you, causing the foot to be stretched in the opposite direction. At the same time lean forward again, guiding the heel towards the centre of the buttock once more, and stretch the whole front of the foot and toes for a few seconds.

At this point, after releasing the final stretch, cross over to your partner's other side, lay their left leg back on the floor, pick up their right leg at the ankle and begin to give knee Shiatsu to the upper leg (as in Step 1, page 79). Repeat all the sequences again, this time giving pressure, stretch and manipulation to your partner's right leg.

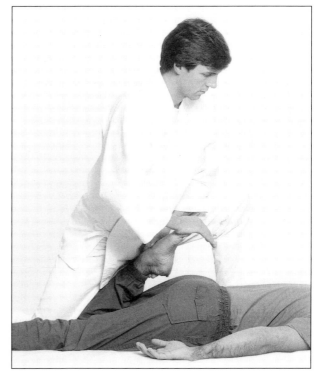

DOUBLE LEG STRETCHES

Do these after completing the final ankle and leg stretch on your partner's right side. They reinforce all the individual leg, ankle and foot work you have just done by giving stretches to both legs at the same time. These sequences also work on the lower back and the fronts of the legs and backs of the thighs.

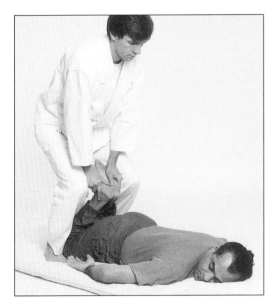

STEP 1 ◄

After finishing the final foot stretch to your partner's right leg, reach round and pick up their left leg, bringing the feet and knees together at right-angles to the floor. Stand up and support both their knees with your insteps on either side, keeping their legs together. Place your palms on their upturned soles, thumbs on the heels and fingers wrapped around the outside of their ankles. Lean down, stretching the Achilles tendon, and then begin leaning forward, bending your knees and guiding their heels towards the centre of their buttocks, stretching the fronts of their legs. Use your whole body in the movement and be sensitive to your partner's maximum stretch point.

STEP 2 ▼ ◄

After releasing the previous stretch, open out your partner's legs by lifting them from the ankles and gently easing them open to a 90° angle. Keep both hands supporting your body weight on their ankles and place one foot on the centre of one of their thighs. Bring the other foot close to the other thigh and, using your palms on their feet to balance yourself, step quickly but gently on to the other thigh.

Your balance is the key to this movement – the moment you feel uncomfortable, step quickly off. Be careful not to place your feet anywhere near the back of the knee.

Once comfortable in this position you can bend your knees, gradually stretching their lower legs forward, heels towards the buttocks as before.

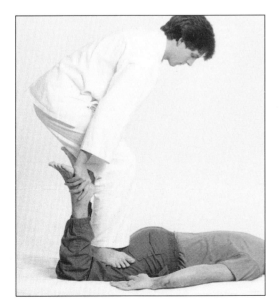

After releasing the final stretch, step off your partner quickly but smoothly and return their feet to the floor, toes pointing in towards each other, heels flopping out, ready for you to walk on their feet . . . .

WALKING ON THE FEET

Strange as it may seem, receiving Shiatsu given with the feet feels comforting and very relaxing. They are a particularly sensitive and perceptive part of our body, and both the giving and receiving of pressure there feels very pleasant.

These sequences are easy to perform and perfectly safe as long as you follow them step by step and don't do any sudden or unexpected movement. But if your partner is unable to turn their toes inwards, or there is too much of a gap between the front of their ankle and the floor, you may have to leave these sequences out. In the latter case you could put a pillow under the fronts of their ankles for support. With elderly people, whose bones are more brittle, just give gentle pressure to one foot at a time.

Balance is a key factor here, as your feet and legs will tend to tense up if you are unsteady. Though imperceptible to you, your partner will easily feel this and will not relax fully. If you need to, find something like a wall to hold on to.

When 'walking', keep your body upright and relaxed just as if you were going for a stroll. Don't step too carefully or timidly – your partner will pick up your hesitancy and again feel less able to relax.

THE BENEFITS

These are much the same as outlined above in all the foot sequences, but here general pressure to the sole of the foot will stimulate functioning of all the internal organs through the reflex areas and meridians. The ankle stretch will especially benefit stiffness and pain in the ankle joints caused by lack of exercise or arthritis.

STEP 1 ▶

Keeping your heels on the ground, place the fronts of your feet over both your partner's insteps and lean your body weight forwards. Alternately shift your body weight from left to right foot as if you were 'walking' on the spot. Stand up straight and keep the rest of your body as loose as you can. Vary the amount of pressure you give by supporting more or less weight on your heels.

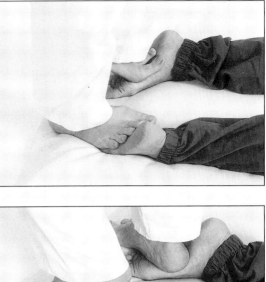

STEP 2 ▼ ▶

Step off your partner's feet, turn round so that your back is facing them and repeat the same movement, this time using your heels instead of the front of your feet to apply the pressure.

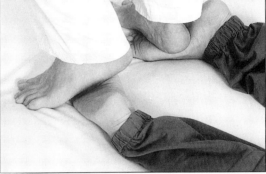

STEP 3 ▼ ▶

After finishing 'walking' on the feet, place one foot across one of your partner's insteps, heel on the sole and front of your foot resting on their inner ankle. Lean your weight forward and gently stretch their ankle open. If you feel your foot position is stable enough, step on to your partner's other foot in the same way so that you are now supporting your whole body weight on the insides of their ankles and feet. Don't move about in this position – just hold it for a few seconds and then step off quickly and smoothly.

Step off your partner's feet and get ready to start the finishing strokes . . . .

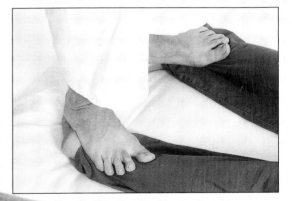

FINISHING STROKES

After completing the last sequence in the prone position, walking on the feet, you are now ready to ask your partner to turn over gently to begin the supine position. However, the following are a series of strokes which allow you to smooth over the work you have done. This type of stroke is less like Shiatsu and more akin to *Anma*, the traditional massage of Japan. Like Western massage it stimulates and invigorates and signals to your partner a change of rhythm and movement, preparing them for a change of position.

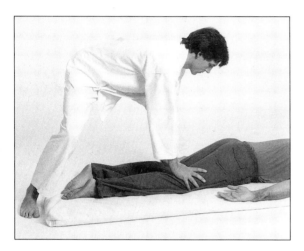

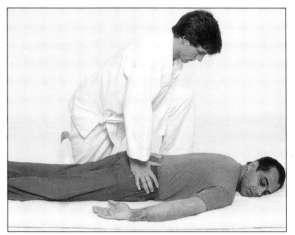

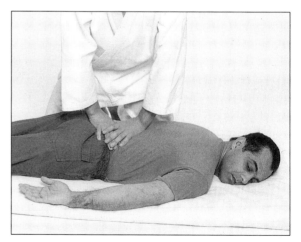

STEP 1 ▲

Stand up and lean forward and down, making contact with your palms on the top of your partner's thighs. In one swift, firm movement 'brush' down your partner's legs several times as far as the feet.

STEP 2 ▲ ▶

Move up to your partner's thighs, kneeling alongside them with your left knee up, foot flat on the floor. Place your palms on both their buttocks at the top near the hips. Using your whole body weight in the movement, firmly and quickly rotate both buttocks in either direction.

STEP 3 ▶ ▲

Move level with your partner's lower back, turning to face them and placing your palms, one over the other, across their spine just above the sacrum. Grip the lower back area gently but firmly with your thumbs on the near side, fingers wrapped around the far side. Again, using your whole body, gently 'rock' your partner back and forth, causing a wave effect to ripple down their whole body.

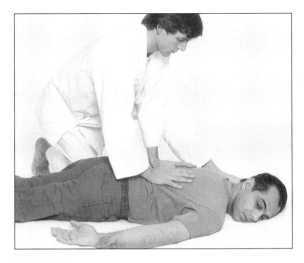

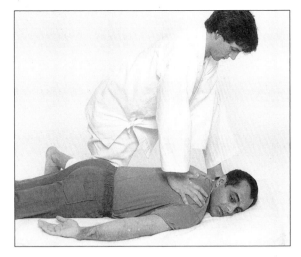

STEP 4 ▲

Turn sideways on to your partner again and move up to your partner's upper back. Place palms either side of the spine and 'brush' down their back from the shoulders to the sacrum, moving your body weight back as you go.

STEP 5 ▲

Move up to your partner's shoulders. Place your palms on top of their shoulder blades and, using your whole body in the movement, rotate the shoulders in both directions.

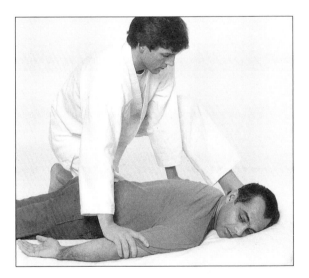

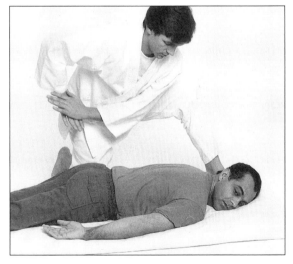

STEP 6 ▲

Place your palms flat on your partner's shoulder blades again and, leaning your body weight backwards, 'brush' down their arms all the way to the hands.

STEP 7 ▶▲

Place your right palm on the top of your partner's back between the shoulder blades, fingers pointing up towards their head, their spine

running under your fingers. Now place your left palm on top of the right one and 'brush' down your partner's spine right the way to the sacrum. This stroke should be firm and invigorating.

After the final finishing stroke, lean forward and whisper to your partner that it is time to turn over gently to lie on their back ready for the supine position . . . .

SUPINE (*Lying on your back*)

Sometimes called the 'corpse' position in Yoga, lying on the back with the feet about shoulder width apart, palms facing up, is probably the easiest position in which to relax completely. When fully calm and at rest the body almost seems to float, which is an ideal state when receiving Shiatsu. Some people, however, if they suffer from backache, may prefer to raise their knees a little.

In this position you can give Shiatsu to some of the most vulnerable areas of the body, especially the lower belly or 'Hara' in Japanese. We need to adjust our pressure as, compared to the other positions, some people can find these areas very sensitive and even uncomfortable.

Because of its extremely relaxing effect, this position is best used at the end of your treatment. Within the series of sequences illustrated in this book I have included it as a natural follow-on from the prone position. In practice, if you have a Shiatsu treatment from a professional practitioner you are likely to be asked to begin in this position for them to palpate your 'Hara' in order to make the initial 'diagnosis' – ie, to establish the primary source of energetic imbalance in the body's organ and meridian systems.

'HARA'

The Japanese word 'Hara' literally means 'belly', though it has the connotation of the centre of one's physical, mental and spiritual being. It is here that the work of digestion is done; it is also the focus of correct breathing, thus concentrating in one area the two main sources of energy available to us – food and oxygen. It houses all the vital organs (except the brain), and in oriental medicine is seen as the root and origin of 'Ki' or vital energy, and of the entire meridian system which distributes it around the body. This is symbolised in the area three fingers' width below the navel, known as 'Tan den', around the point 'Ki kai', which means 'sea of Ki' or vital energy.

In oriental medicine, the relationship between good health and a strong 'Hara' is an accepted fact. The practice of Shiatsu itself requires 'Hara' (movement from the centre), and the abdomen is used to diagnose and treat conditions which affect the whole body. In Japan, 'Ampuka' therapy is the art of diagnosing and treating illness from the 'Hara' alone.

We should think of it as representing the very roots of our being, which need special care for the rest of us to be able to thrive.

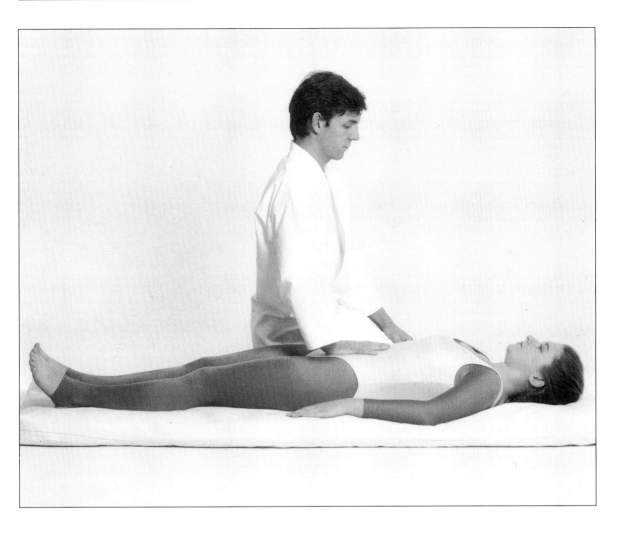

STEP 1 ▲

In dealing with such a key area of the body, it will take all your concentration and attention to make your first contact with your partner's abdomen convey warmth and reassurance. You must be at your most relaxed and yet most alert, completely tuned in to your partner before even attempting contact. Sit alongside them, your right thigh in contact with the side of their body, until you feel ready to begin. Slowly bring your right palm down on to the centre of their abdomen, at first touching very lightly and gradually, but gently leaning over to your side to apply soft pressure on to your palm. Hold this position for as long as you feel comfortable,

following their breathing and allowing them to relax after having turned over from the prone position.

STEP 2

In your own time, begin gently wiping down their abdomen from top to bottom with both your palms in a gentle brushing movement. Try to visualise the energy moving down to their legs.

When you are ready, turn to face your partner level with their hips and get ready to begin palm shiatsu to the legs . . .

LEG STRETCHES AND PRESSURE

Having worked on both of the legs in the prone position, you can now give pressure and stretches to the fronts of the legs, reaching all the remaining areas. Here you can again alter your partner's leg position to reach different lines to work on, so that your own position can remain stable throughout. However, because you are now dealing with softer and more vulnerable areas you use the palms instead of the knees to apply pressure.

The main feature of these sequences is that they provide stretch and pressure in the same position. The only change from one to the other is the position of the support hand. This is always placed in the most comfortable position over the protruding part of the front of the pelvis (anterior ileac crest), part of the palm on the bone, part on the lower abdomen. If pressure is applied to the opposite leg to where the support hand is, a stretch will occur; if on the same side, only pressure will be given. To stretch, you must give double-handed pressure and rock back and forth to release and apply it with each hand on opposite sides of your partner. When both hands are on the same side, pressure is applied in the usual way by shifting from support hand to giving hand until equalised, without rocking your body.

THE BENEFITS

On page 78 I mentioned the many symptoms typically found in the legs. This is partly due to insufficient use and partly because we often fail to use our 'Hara' in daily activity and movement. In walking, sitting and generally moving about we tend to over-emphasise our upper bodies.

These sequences continue the work of encouraging proper 'Ki' blood and fluid flow through the legs, begun in the prone position. They allow us to reach the three leg Yin meridians – liver, kidney and spleen which, in oriental medicine, play a large part in the function of manufacturing, transporting, storing and releasing the blood.

Pressure here is useful in treating poor circulation, cramps, weakness in the legs and oedema (water-retention), and it can help regulate menstrual problems such as cramping, irregular, painful or heavy periods, and pre-menstrual tension in general.

The stretches open up the whole pelvic area as well as the meridians and are helpful for libido problems as well as frigidity, tension and pain in the inner thighs.

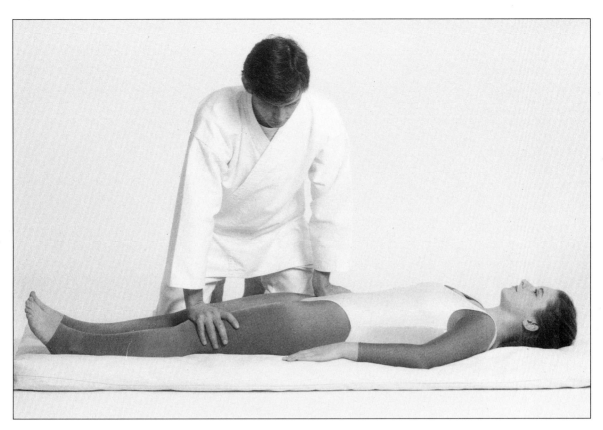

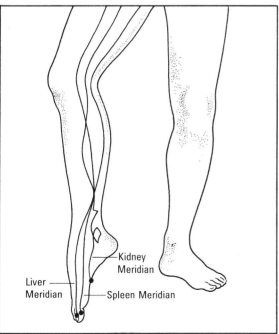

Kidney
Meridian

Liver
Meridian

Spleen Meridian

STEP 1 ▲

After finishing palming over the 'Hara', turn to face your partner, kneeling, level with their thighs. As in the prone position, make sure you can reach the feet without over-reaching yourself; you may need to shift your position. Place your left hand over the bony part of the front of your partner's pelvis, so that the centre of your palm is on the bone and your fingers on the lower abdomen. Make sure you find a comfortable position for your partner to take your weight – this area can be very sensitive. With your right hand, give palm Shiatsu down the far leg from hip to toes twice.

STEP 2

When palming down the near leg, turn the palm in the opposite direction, fingers facing towards you, heel facing away, and repeat the same movement as in Step 1.

STEP 3 ▶

Turn the near (right) foot in, so that the sole faces the opposite ankle and the knee is bent, exposing the inside of the near leg. Now give palm pressure to the first of three lines (see the diagram on page 95) along the inside of the leg down to the foot. With the support hand on the far hip you can give stretches; moving it to the near hip will allow you to give full pressure.

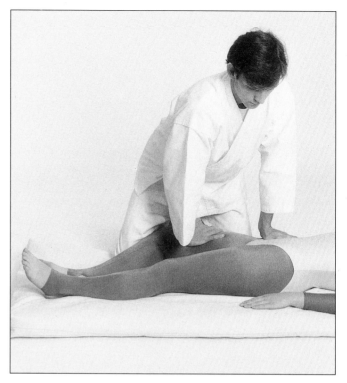

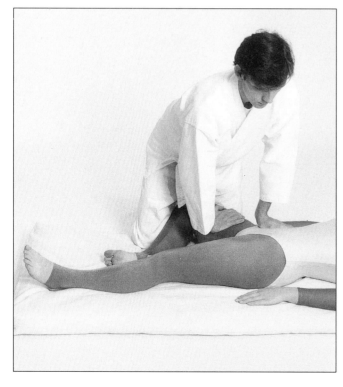

STEP 4 ◀

Slide your partner's right foot up level with their opposite knee so that the near leg makes a right-angle. Now give stretch and pressure to the second line along the leg as far as the foot. Repeat this twice, moving the support hand to the far side for the stretch and the near side to apply pressure.

STEP 5 ▶

Finally, slide your partner's foot right up so that the heel moves up towards the groin and their right leg is fully bent, with the calf touching the back of their thigh. Now give stretch and pressure to the third line along the inside of the leg, moving the support hand from hip to hip as before.

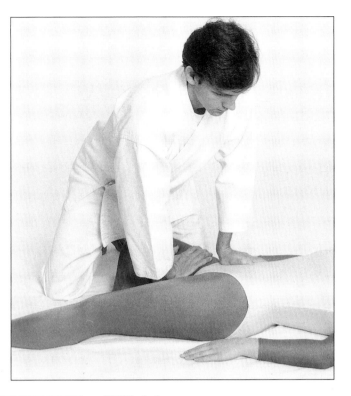

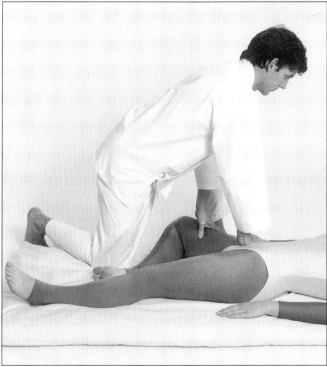

STEP 6 ◀

To give more specific pressure to each of the three lines, you can use your thumb, following the same sequences as in Steps 3–5. Begin with the stretches in each position as before but, to apply the pressure, place the thumb in position on the chosen line, fingers wrapped around the thigh. Lean in, transferring the weight from support hand to giving hand.

Kneel up, taking your partner's right foot in your right hand and tucking your left forearm under the back of their knee. Step out with your left foot, keeping your right knee on the ground, and get ready to give the leg and hip stretches and rotations. . . .

LEG AND HIP STRETCHES AND ROTATIONS

Having completed your pressure work on the leg, you can now stretch and manipulate the whole limb. Because of the size and weight of the leg itself, you must use your whole body in the movement to avoid the need for strength. Maintain maximum contact with your partner by holding their leg close to your chest, and coordinate the movement of your shoulder and knee to give smooth, effortless movement from the hips. In this way your hands become merely guiding influences to alter the direction of the stretch or rotation. You should not rely on them to initiate the movement, otherwise you will find it a struggle – especially with a tall partner who has long, heavy legs. Ideally you should be able to manipulate your partner's leg without effort, no matter what the size or weight.

THE BENEFITS

When 'Ki' gets blocked or stuck its effects are often felt most acutely in the joints. This is because, as mentioned before, 'Ki', blood and fluids flow abundantly in the joint cavities. Therefore, after freeing up and balancing 'Ki' flow in the leg meridians with the stretch and pressure you have already done, you must loosen the hip joint and make sure proper flow is maintained with the rest of the body. These rotations and stretches improve flexibility by restoring proper 'Ki' and blood flow to the area, helping relieve problems like arthritis, cramps, sciatica, numbness, poor circulation and tiredness and heaviness in the legs.

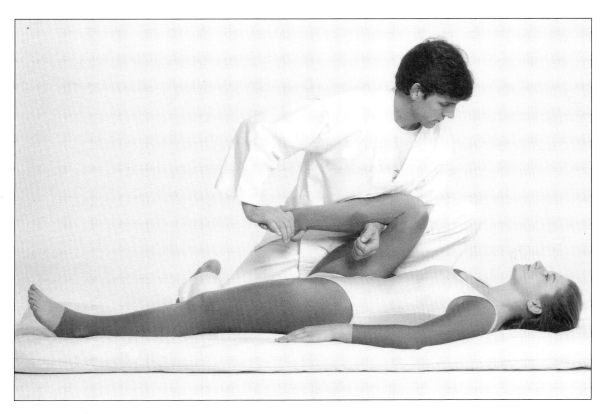

STEP 1 ▲

After finishing palm and thumb pressure to the third line on the inside of the leg, kneel up, taking your partner's right foot in your right hand and tucking your left forearm under the back of their right knee. Step up and out with your left foot, keeping your right knee on the ground, and lean forward, stretching your partner's leg, knee towards their chest. Your left hand should be relaxed, your right loosely holding your partner's foot and helping to guide the leg forward. The stretch comes entirely from the weight of your body leaning forward. Drop your left shoulder as you lean, and coordinate the movement of this shoulder with your left knee. Repeat the stretch several times, moving your left forearm gradually down the back of your partner's thigh.

STEP 2

Following the stretch, begin to rotate the leg in a clockwise direction, starting with small circles and gradually getting bigger until maximum rotation is reached. Do this by moving your whole upper body from the waist and guiding your partner's knee around with your left knee and shoulder. Then repeat the movement anti-clockwise. As with the arm rotations in the sitting position (see page 42), don't force the movement. If your partner resists, try loosening the joint by shaking the leg a little before rotating.

Release your partner's leg and gently lower it back to the floor in the straight position. Step back with the left leg, placing the left knee on the floor, and step up with the right leg, placing the right foot on the floor just beyond your partner's feet. Cup your right hand under your partner's right heel and get ready to give the full leg stretches....

FULL LEG STRETCHES

These stretches complete the series of sequences for each leg individually and are followed by the double-leg sequences. They are somewhat similar to the single leg stretches done in the prone position, though here the leg is straight rather than bent.

Here the body weight is used like a lever in both directions to give the stretches, and the support hand is used to fix the leg in position and prevent it from lifting and rolling from side to side.

It is vital not to use muscle power in giving the stretches – it will make your partner tense and exhaust you! You will also be less sensitive to how far to take the stretch. Keep your arms loose, and use them rather as levers which are controlled by the movement of your body and cannot act independently of it.

THE BENEFITS

These stretches mainly benefit the ankle and toe joints, improving flexibility and stimulating 'Ki' and blood flow to the area. As mentioned before, stiffness in the ankles and toes impairs proper meridian function and can lead to stagnation in the whole leg. In oriental medicine flexible, healthy toes, like the fingers, are considered very important to one's general health.

These stretches also work on the urinary bladder and stomach meridians – the one related to the back of the legs, the other to the front.

Overall, the stretches can help relieve cramps, numbness, pain and mobility problems caused by stagnation and blockage of energy, blood and fluid circulation, as well as by weakness.

STEP 1 ▶

After finishing the leg rotations and returning the leg to the floor in the straight position, shift your left foot back so that you are momentarily kneeling on both knees. Then step out with your right foot, placing it beyond your partner's feet. Cup your right hand under the heel of their right foot, grasping the heel with your fingers and allowing your palm and wrist to rest on the sole of their foot. Now lean your body weight directly away from their feet, up towards their head, moving from your hips. To prevent their whole leg rising off the ground and to support your body weight, place your left hand just above their right knee and lean down on to it.

STEP 2 ▼▶

Keep your support (left) hand where it is and release the right hand from the sole of your partner's foot, placing it on top of the foot, your fingers over their toes. Now shift your body weight in the opposite direction as in Step 1, away from your partner's head, towards their feet, stretching the toes towards the floor. Get your body weight over the top of your partner's foot so you can just lean down over it – don't use any strength to give the stretch.

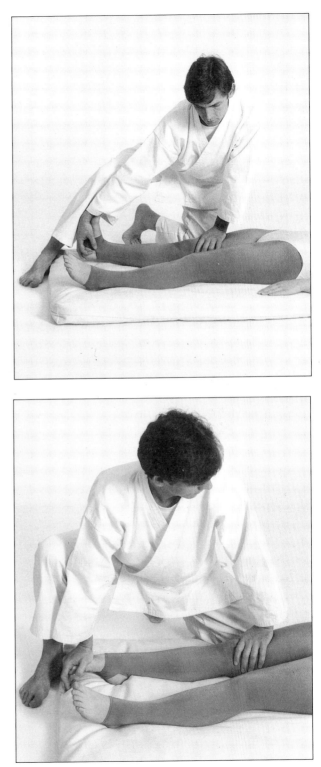

Now you have finished working on your partner's near (right) leg. Cross over to the opposite side, maintaining contact with your partner, and position yourself as before. Kneeling with your giving hand (left) ready to work on the first of the three leg lines. Repeat all the above sequences from page 95, this time working on your partner's left leg.

When you have completed the last sequence (i.e. the full leg stretch) move round to kneel at your partner's feet, facing their head. Take hold of their ankles, cupping them behind the heels with your palm. Lean gently backwards, ready to give the double leg stretch. . . .

STEP 1

After finishing the final leg stretch to your partner's left leg, move round to the feet and, kneeling to face their head, take hold of both their ankles, supporting at the back of the heel with your palms. Now simply lean your body weight back and, with straight arms, apply a full leg stretch equally to the left and right side together. Watch your partner's head and you should see it move slightly as the stretch is felt through the whole body up to the neck. Apply and release the stretch slowly and evenly.

Now replace one leg on the floor, placing your knee under the sole of the foot. Keep hold of your partner's other leg at the ankle and get ready to give the single leg pressure, stretches and rotations. . . .

DOUBLE LEG STRETCH

Having worked on the legs individually, now you can work on both legs simultaneously. This is done to balance the left and right sides as well as to check any differences between them. For example, you may notice that one is longer than the other or simply that one is looser or stiffer. This may determine whether you choose to go back and work more on one of the legs.

In this movement your grip is important. Don't grasp the ankles too tightly – this may stretch the skin and cause pain. Simply cup the heels in the palms of your hands and lean back. Because your arms are angled upwards, giving some lift to your movement, the heels will not slide out of your palms and you won't have to hold them tightly at all.

The other feature of this movement is to let yourself lean naturally backwards, without checking yourself by using your muscles. The weight of your partner's body will stop you and allow a comfortable stretch without you having to pull or use your strength. Your arms should be straight, not locked and relaxed.

THE BENEFITS

Much the same as for the single leg stretches, this movement benefits energy, blood and fluid circulation to the whole leg area, relieving the same kinds of problem. It also has a balancing effect on the meridian energy left and right, as well as releasing tension and blockage in the joints and pelvis. Done correctly, the stretch will be felt all the way up the spine and has the effect of relieving compression and blocked energy in the vertebrae – acting as a kind of traction. This is excellent for the relief of back and neck ache caused by bad posture, tension or injury.

FOOT PRESSURE, STRETCHES AND ROTATIONS

Any work on the legs would be incomplete without attending to the ankles and feet. It is they that carry our full body weight for most of our waking hours, and we are dependent on their strength and flexibility to move around. Many people have problems with their feet, caused by bad posture, ill-fitting shoes and lack of exercise. A tendency to stand with more weight on one foot than the other, or with the weight poorly distributed (for example as a result of wearing high-heeled shoes), or simply failing to exercise the area, especially the toes, can result in cramps, stiffness and rheumatic pains in the joints, as well as walking difficulties.

These simple sequences stretch and rotate all the joints of the foot and can be used as a mini-treatment in themselves – everyone loves having their feet touched! The movements are quite straightforward. If you partner stiffens or resists the movements, simply shake the foot and leg to loosen them.

THE BENEFITS

Since the feet can carry a great deal of tension, working to relieve this and to restore proper energy flow in the local area can have a strong effect on the whole body. Structurally, there are many bones and muscles in the feet, any one of which can get tense or slightly out of position, causing cramps and stiffness and affecting movement. We may then favour one particular foot when walking, and this 'one-sidedness' can quickly cause more widespread imbalance in the body posture as a whole. Keeping the feet strong and flexible is therefore essential to good health.

In oriental medicine, as I have mentioned earlier, there are reflex areas on the sole of the foot related to different parts of the body, including the internal organs. This enables you to work from this area and affect the whole body. Also, as in the hands, main meridians start and finish in the toes, so that flexibility of the joints and muscles is vital to maintaining proper flow through the whole meridian system. Cramped, twisted and inflexible toes can impair the free flow of 'Ki' in the meridians, causing other imbalances throughout the body.

STEP 1

After the double leg stretch replace your partner's left leg on the floor, placing your right knee under the sole of their foot. Keep their right ankle cupped in the palm of your left hand and place your right hand over the back of their toes. In one movement lean back, stretching their leg towards you with your left hand and pressing their toes away from you with your right, stretching the sole of the foot and Achilles tendon.

Releasing the foot stretch with the right hand but maintaining the leg stretch with the left, place your right palm over the front of the toes and stretch the foot down towards the ground, using your body weight to lean over and down.

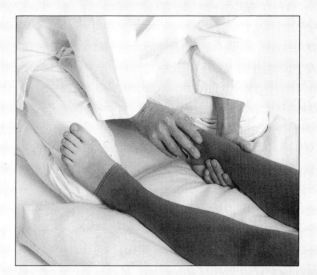

STEP 2 ▶

Now that your partner's right foot is back on the floor, keep your support (left) hand at the ankle and bring your right hand to join it. Using your thumbs, give pressure to the lines on top of the foot (see the diagram). Give plenty of support with one hand while applying pressure with the thumb of the other, wrapping the fingers around the sole of the foot for extra support.

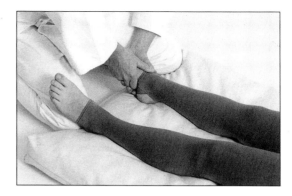

STEP 3 ▼ ▶

Now bring your partner's foot up on to your left knee so that the sole of the foot is facing you. Take the whole foot firmly in both hands, wrapping your fingers around the top of the foot and allowing both thumbs to rest on the sole. Lean your body weight forward and apply pressure along the lines shown in the diagram, paying particular attention to the point shown.

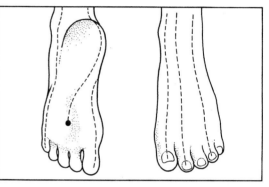

STEP 4 ▼ ▶

Keeping the left hand supporting the heel, lean forward and drop your left forearm on to your left knee, resting your body weight on it. Now, still cupping your partner's right ankle in your left palm, begin to rotate the foot with your right hand. Make big, fluent rotations in both directions, keeping the ankle firmly supported in your left hand.

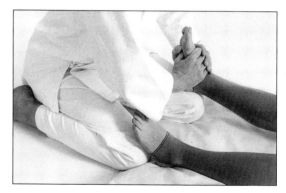

Now replace the foot on the floor, shift your left knee to support the sole of your partner's right foot and pick up their left leg in your right hand, supporting it at the ankle. Repeat Steps 1–4 above to their right foot. Then replace the leg on the floor, bring both their feet together and secure them between your knees, ready to give pressure, stretches and rotations to the legs, toes and ankles. . . .

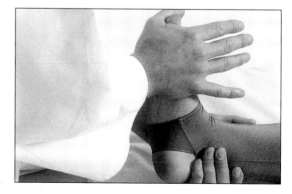

DOUBLE LEG, ANKLE & TOE PRESSURE, STRETCH & ROTATION

STEP 1 ▶

After finishing the pressure, stretch and rotation to each leg individually, bring your partner's legs together, supporting their feet between your knees. Kneel up and lean over their lower legs, making a loose fist with both hands. Now place the fist at the top of the shin bone below the knee – thumbs on the insides of the bone, fingers on the outsides. Lean your body weight down, applying pressure gradually down the whole lower leg on both sides simultaneously as far as the ankle.

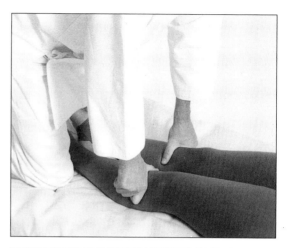

STEP 2 ▶ ▼

Sit back on to your heels again and, using your thumbs and forefingers, grasp each toe individually in turn, gently squeezing, stretching and rotating them. Finally, give each a gentle lift, so that the heels rise a little off the floor and the natural weight of the foot itself gives a stretch to each toe in turn.

STEP 3 ▶ ▼

Place your palms over the underside of the toes and, with your elbows held into your chest, lean forward and rock their feet gently back and forth. This will create a wave-like rocking movement throughout the body; you can vary the strength and speed by using your body weight.

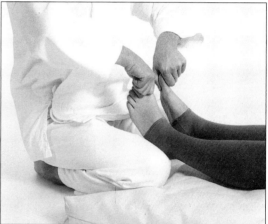

STEP 4

Open your knees wide, gently separating your partner's feet again. Now rotate the feet inwards so the toes point in towards each other. Begin to make small, rhythmic, circular movements with your palms, again sending a rocking movement right through your partner's body, similar to Step 3.

Bring your partner's feet together again, grasping the heels with both hands. Come up on to your feet in the squatting position and, with straight arms, lean back to give a double leg stretch....

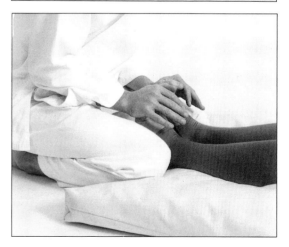

DOUBLE LEG STRETCH, SHAKE AND SWAY

This stretch is very similar to that shown on page 102, except that here you are squatting rather than kneeling. The benefits are the same.

The squatting position is important to the next sequence, which involves standing up, using your partner's 'dead weight' to counter-balance yourself as you push upwards in one smooth movement. (This change of position would involve two separate movements from the kneeling position.)

The use of your partner's weight literally to pull yourself up into the standing position is repeated later in the supine position (see page 141), in that case using their arms instead of their legs. Again, this avoids the need for any effort on your part and maintains flow and rhythm in your movement.

When standing to give the shake and sway, make sure your own position is stable and comfortable. Bend your knees a little to ease any unnecessary pressure on the lower back. When you make the movements, use your whole body and not just your hands or arms. Sometimes your partner may stiffen at the hips, especially during the sway. Adopt your usual tactics of gently shaking the limbs to loosen them up before trying the movement again.

THE BENEFITS

This series of sequences helps to loosen the joints of the legs, especially the hips. In performing the sway, you should get the legs to move in a wide arc so that maximum movement of the hip joint is achieved. A lot of people carry tension in their pelvis and hips, and loosening up this area can be very effective in releasing overall body tension. People are so used to consciously moving their own legs that to have them manipulated by someone else is often strange at first, and it may be difficult simply to 'let go'. But when they do, they will feel a tremendous sense of lightness and release.

STEP 1 ▼

Having finished rocking the body from the feet, bring your partner's feet together and, holding the ankles in your palms, come up on to your feet in the squatting position. Now simply lean backwards, allowing your body weight to stretch your partner from the legs. This is similar to the stretch on page 102.

Having completed the double leg stretch, keep leaning backwards and, maintaining the stretch, push upwards with your legs, thrusting your body weight up into the standing position. The further backwards you lean your body, the less power you will need actually to stand up....

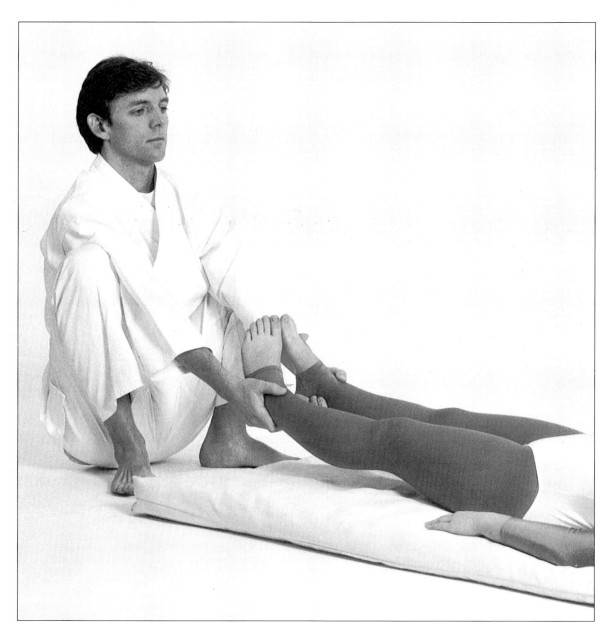

STEP 2
In the standing position, feet shoulder width apart, knees bent, back straight, begin to shake your partner's legs alternately from the ankles. Make the movement as natural and loose as possible, so that any stiffness is released from their legs and they become jelly-like.

STEP 3 ▼

Step wider with your feet, maintaining your grip at the back of your partner's ankles. Begin to sway your upper body from side to side, using your hips rather than your arms to control the movement. Let the arms follow, and with them your partner's legs, so that you begin swaying them from side to side quite vigorously. Try not to move their upper body – the movement should come from their hips.

After finishing the final sway bring your feet together again, placing the soles of your partner's feet on your knees. Now walk forward, guiding their knees towards their chest with your hands, ready to give a stretch....

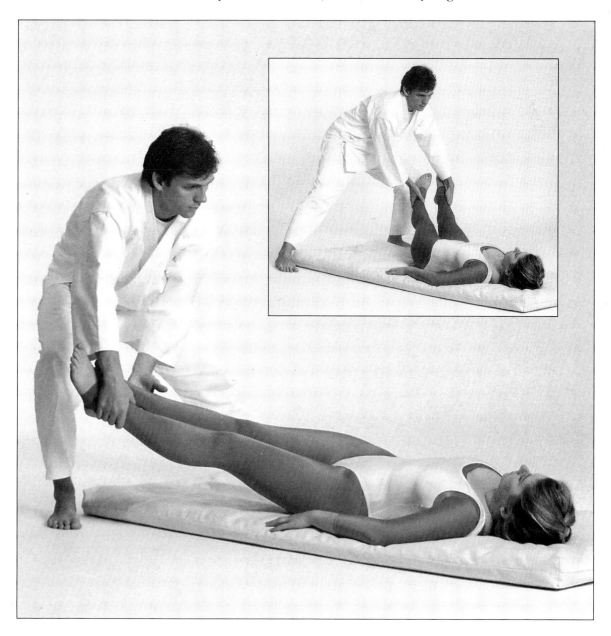

HIP STRETCHES AND ROTATIONS AND LEG WIPE

Here are the final leg sequences before moving up to work on the arms. Movement of the hips and pelvis was not possible to any great degree in the prone position, so these sequences are especially important to include in your total body treatment. Pay attention to your standing posture, as you don't want to put unnecessary strain on your back. Keeping your centre of gravity low by bending the knees and dropping the hips is invariably the most stable and comfortable position for these movements.

The first two positions, (Steps 1 and 2), are relatively straight-forward, though care should be taken with older or less flexible people. Simply make smaller and more gentle movements and don't lean down too heavily.

With the last position (Step 3) it is essential not to overstretch your partner. Just take them gently to their maximum stretch point and, as with all the stretches, simply hold it for a few seconds before releasing. Never 'bounce' or force the stretch further. Pay attention to the position of the support hand, which should be placed on the front of the shoulder not on the shoulder joint itself (see Step 3).

THE BENEFITS

These sequences help improve flexibility in the hip joints, pelvis and lower back. In Western exercise systems a great deal of emphasis is placed on cardio-vascular fitness, with movements designed to work on the upper body, heart and lungs. Many oriental systems, however, including the martial arts and Yoga, tend to concentrate on opening up and strengthening the body's natural centre, which encompasses the lower abdomen, hips and pelvis. This area is thought of as a vital centre from which energy is directed outwards in all directions to the four limbs. Maintaining strength and flexibility here through movements like this is therefore seen as essential to one's overall health.

STEP 1 ▶

After finishing the double leg sway, bring your own and your partner's feet together, placing their soles on your knees. Now walk forward, guiding their knees to their chest with your hands. Use your body weight to lean over and down towards their chest, pressing on their knees with your palms and pushing the soles of their feet forward with your knees until they reach their natural stretch point. Hold this position for a few seconds before releasing.

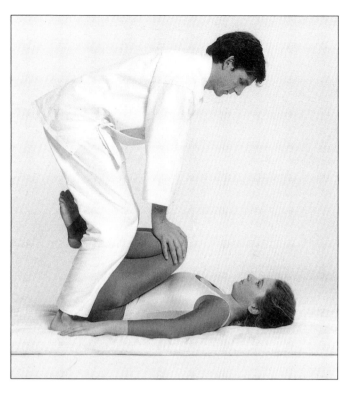

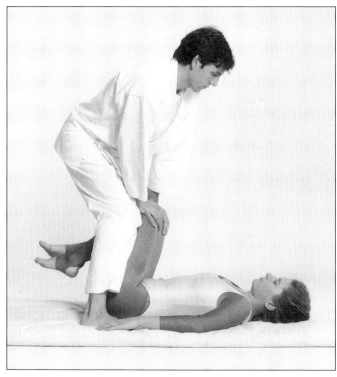

STEP 2 ◀

Release your partner's knees from their chest and bring them up into a vertical position, securing them between your knees. Keeping your palms on top of their knees, begin to make large rotating movements using your pelvis and knees. Rotate their knees and pelvis in both directions, increasing the size of the circles as appropriate. Use your whole body, not just your knees.

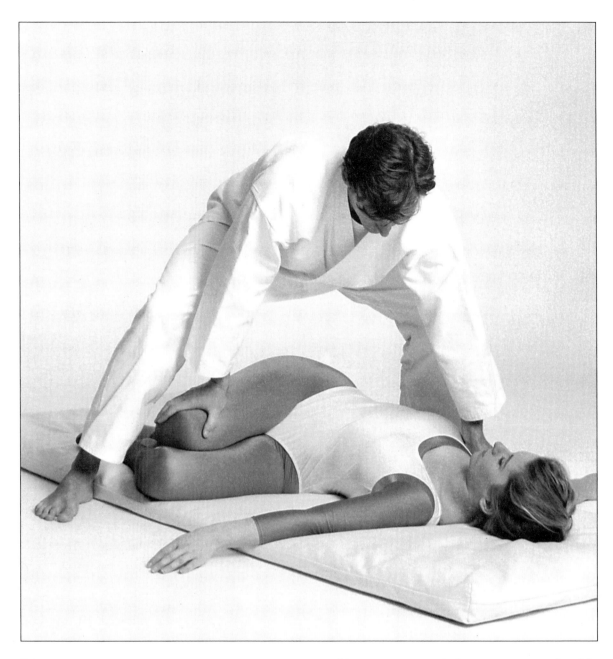

STEP 3 ▲

Take a step to the side with your right foot, keeping your partner's knees vertical with your right hand. Lean forward and place your left palm on the front of their right shoulder. Bending your knees and keeping your weight low, gradually lean over to your right, gently pushing your partner's knees across to the side with your right hand until they touch the floor. Maintain equal pressure on both of your hands. Naturally, if a stretch occurs before your partner's knees touch the floor, don't force the movement any further. Repeat the stretch to the other side.

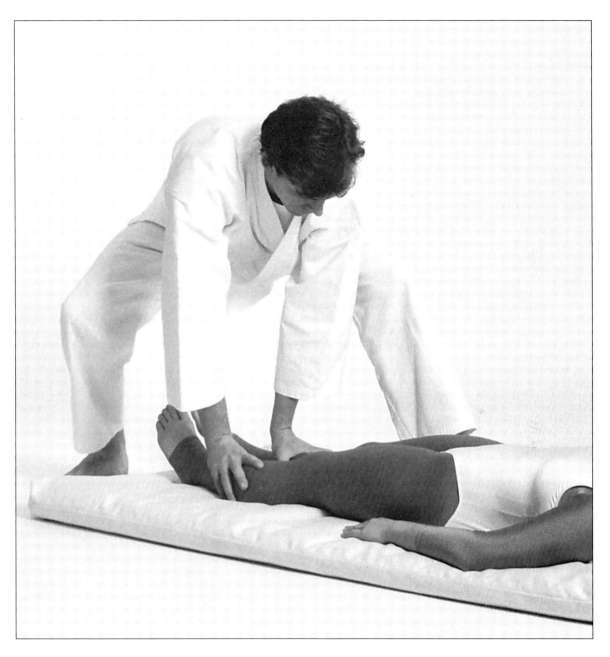

STEP 4 ▲

After finishing Step 3 on both sides, take hold of your partner's ankles, step back and gently lower their legs to the floor. Now step alongside their legs and, leaning over and down, brush firmly down both legs from hips to toes. Repeat this movement several times.

Having completed your work on the legs, move up level with the shoulders and, kneeling, open your partner's arm out to the side, palm up, ready for you to give pressure to the arms....

ARMS (PRESSURE)

In the prone position you have already done some work 'walking' down the arms with your palms. In these sequences, too, you can use palm pressure, though elbow pressure is used to be more specific to the meridians.

The most important aspect of this sequence is the location of the support hand. This must be placed on the front of the shoulder – on the top of the chest, in effect – and not on the shoulder joint, which is painful when pressure is applied. As usual, pressure must be distributed equally between both hands. As with the knee joint, the elbow joint does not bear pressure well and you should avoid resting your body weight directly on it.

When using your elbows, the movement is very similar to giving knee Shiatsu to the back of the leg in the prone position (page 79). First the upper limb is worked on, with the support below the joint, and then the lower limb, changing hands and supporting above the joint.

Don't hang back with your hips, but kneel right up so that your full body weight is available to apply the pressure.

THE BENEFITS

As with the legs, proper flow of 'Ki', blood and body fluids to the arms is vital for healthy balance in the body's systems as a whole. Though we are two-legged animals now, and have developed other uses for our arms, they were clearly used for locomotion originally, as they still are when we are babies.

Shiatsu maintains proper energy flow in the arm meridians, preventing numbness, cramps, pain and stiffness, whilst the stretches and rotations help improve and maintain flexibility in the joints. Naturally, this has a knock-on effect and helps keep the shoulders looser also. These sequences particularly benefit the three arm Yin meridians (lung, heart and heart constrictor), which affect circulation of energy and blood.

STEP 1 ▶

Having moved up level with the shoulders after completing work on the legs, open out your partner's right arm to the side, palm upwards. Kneel up and place your right palm on the front of your partner's right shoulder at the top of their chest. Now begin palming down the arm from shoulder to fingers, transferring your body weight from one side to the other in the usual way.

STEP 2 ▼

After palming down the arm, place your left hand as support just below your partner's elbow joint. Taking your body weight here, position your right forearm ready to give pressure to the upper arm from the armpit to the elbow. Work down three lines in turn, following the lung, heart constrictor and heart meridians respectively (see pages 16–17). Work on each line twice.

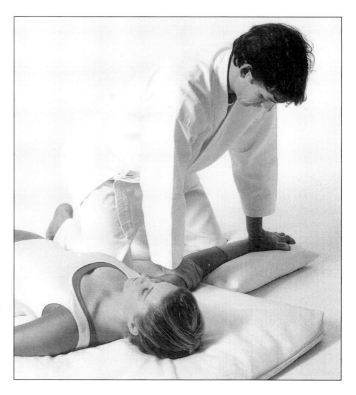

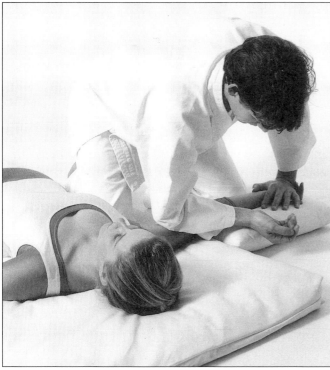

STEP 3

Now place your right hand as support just above the elbow joint. Take your body weight here and position your left forearm ready to give pressure to your partner's forearm from the elbow to the wrist. Follow the same three lines as in Step 2, repeating each line twice.

Now take hold of your partner's right wrist with your left hand. Move your right hand support to their shoulder joint and, stepping forward with your left foot, get ready to do the arm rotations....

ARM ROTATIONS, STRETCHES AND SHAKE

Once again, following pressure work to an area – in this case the shoulder joint and arm – we can stretch and manipulate it. This movement is similar to the arm rotation in the sitting position (see page 43), except that here the support hand is placed on the front of the shoulder rather than on the back. Good support to the shoulder joint during the rotation is important to enable a stretch to be maintained through the movement. Equally important is the use of your body weight to direct and control the movement of your partner's arm – don't use your strength. The arm rotation should look similar to a backstroke swimming movement, with as wide an arc as possible taking into account the range of your partner's flexibility. Never force the rotation.

THE BENEFITS

Flexibility of the shoulder joint is vital for proper flow of energy up to the neck and head as well as down the arms. I have already mentioned that the major joint cavities are areas where 'Ki' and blood flow abundantly, so that if they stagnate due to injury, lack of exercise or cold, damp weather, problems such as pain, stiffness, numbness, cramps and cold may arise. Maintaining flexibility in the shoulder joint as well as stimulating the flow of energy in the arm meridians, especially the three arm Yang meridians which run up to the head (large intestine, small intestine, triple heater) will help to combat headaches, stiff neck and shoulders, arthritis and neuralgia in the arms, numbness and tingling in the fingers, poor circulation and cramps.

STEP 1 ▶

After giving pressure down your partner's arm from shoulder to palm, take hold of their right wrist in your left hand and move your right hand to give support at their shoulder joint. In the same movement, step forward with your left foot and bring their arm up against your chest into a stretch.

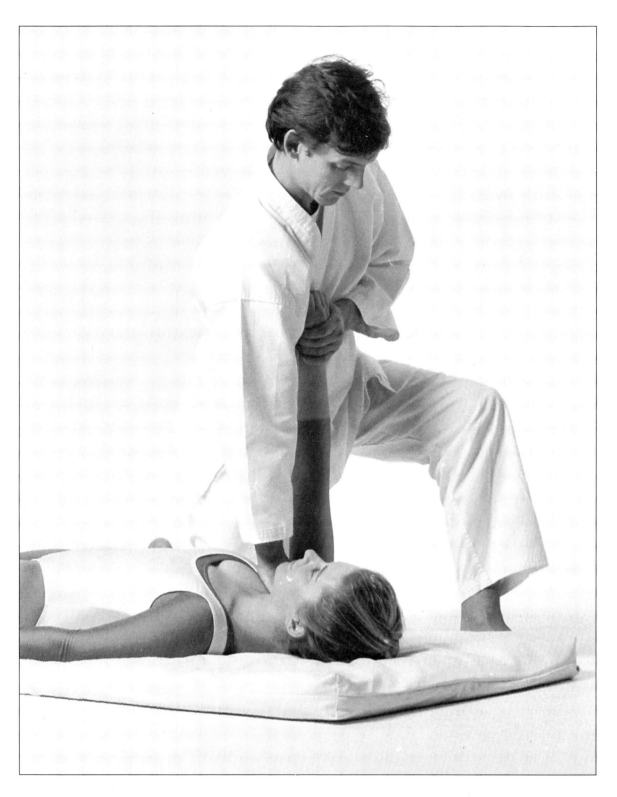

STEP 2

Now begin to make big backward rotations with their arm, like a backstroke movement. Maintain good support with your right hand, using your body weight to control the movement: shifting it back and forth to guide the direction of the arm. Don't use your strength to manipulate the arm, and avoid grasping the wrist too tightly with your left hand.

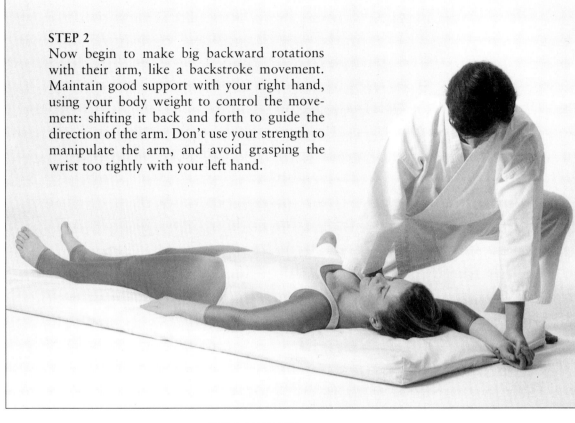

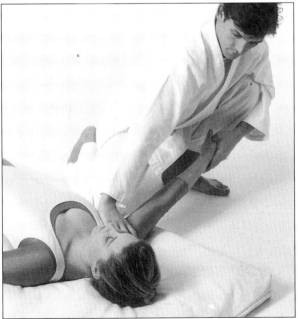

STEP 3 ◄

Keeping hold of your partner's right hand, grasping their fingers with your left hand, tuck the thumb of your right hand under their armpit, wrapping your fingers around the front of their shoulder. In the same movement step away to the side, hooking your left knee inside your left elbow and leaning away from your partner. Holding their shoulder firmly with your right hand, stretch and shake the arm vigorously to the side.

Now release your support (right) hand, keeping hold of your partner's wrist in your left hand, and come to stand level with their shoulder, one foot supporting their upper arm on the floor, ready to work on the palms, fingers and wrist....

PALM, FINGERS AND WRIST STRETCH AND MANIPULATION

There are a number of different methods you can use to work on the hands. These may involve simply laying your partner's hands on your knee and working on them in the kneeling or sitting position. Here I have shown how to work on the hands from the standing position, partly because it is easier to move into the following position from standing, and partly because you can lean your body weight down effortlessly from that position. However, if you find this position uncomfortable simply kneel, hold your partner's hand in your lap and follow the same sequences. The two main points to remember in the standing position are to bend your knees to take any strain off your back, and gently to hold the front of one foot on your partner's upper arm to stop it rising off the floor. When you stretch the fingers, don't lean too heavily on this foot.

THE BENEFITS

As with the feet and toes, flexibility of the hands and fingers is considered a vital sign of good general health in the East. In China, many older people go around constantly rotating two metal balls in one hand, which requires great coordination and dexterity. As previously mentioned, six of the body's twelve meridians begin or end in the fingers, and so there is a great deal of energetic activity here. Maintaining flexibility in the hands and fingers therefore encourages healthy flow of 'Ki' and blood through the meridians, helping prevent stiffness, pain and poor circulation.

STEP 1 ▼

After finishing the arm stretch and shake, come to stand level with your partner's shoulder, holding their right wrist in both your hands and bending the arm at the elbow so that you are holding the forearm vertical with the upper arm still on the floor. Now place the front of your right foot gently on the upper arm and lean a little weight on it to prevent it moving about. Grasping the wrist in both your hands, bend it over, palm towards the ground, and lean your body weight gently down to give a wrist stretch.

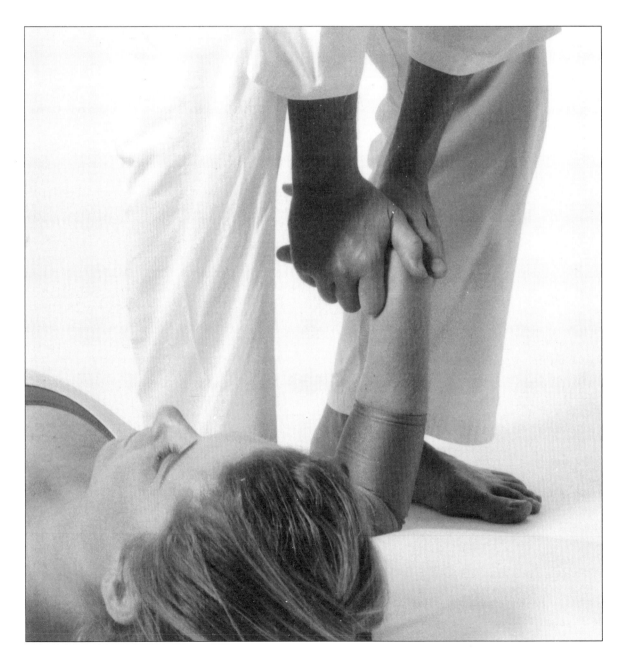

STEP 2 ▶

Release the stretch and bend the wrist back the other way, palm facing up. Now interlock the web of your little fingers between your partner's little and ring fingers on one side and thumb and forefinger on the other, stretching open the palm and pressing your thumb down to give Shiatsu on the palm itself.

STEP 3

Release the palm and, taking the wrist in both hands again, give wrist rotations in both directions, using your whole body in the movement.

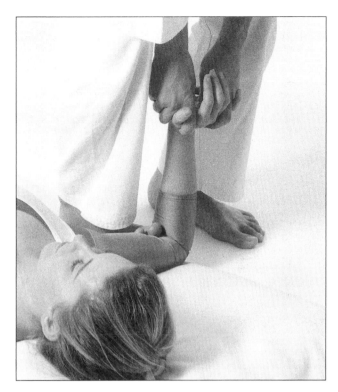

STEP 4 ▶

Now, supporting your partner's wrist with your left hand, with your right begin squeezing and pulling each finger in turn between your index and middle fingers. Don't use the strength of your arm as you pull, but gently raise your body weight slightly to achieve the stretch. Often the fingers will 'crack', but don't deliberately try to make this happen.

After finishing the finger stretches, shake your partner's arm and replace it on the floor. Maintaining contact with one hand, slowly walk over or around their feet to reach the other side. Now repeat the sequences from Step 1 on page 117, this time working on your partner's left arm. When you have finished both arms, move above your partner's head into the kneeling position. Cup your hands behind their neck, ready to give a spine stretch....

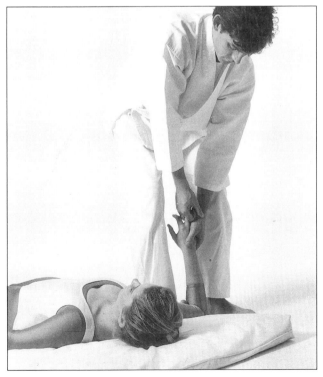

SPINE STRETCH

The effect of this stretch is similar to the one in the prone position (see page 68), except that here it is done from the neck rather than the sacrum.

The neck is one of the most delicate areas to manipulate, and you must take care not to make any sudden or abrupt movements when working on it. The spine stretch is achieved through a combination of firm support with both palms at the base of the skull and a leaning back movement with the rest of the body. Once again the arms are straight and act only as levers – no muscle power is used to actively pull the neck towards you.

The distance you sit from your partner depends on the length of your arms, so adjust your position so that you are neither cramped nor over-stretched. The part of your hand which does most of the support is the little finger edge of the palm, and this area should mould itself to the occipital bone (base of the skull). If you are right-handed, you will find it easier to cup the right hand in the left.

THE BENEFITS

This movement is a form of simple traction which relieves the pain caused by compression of the spine due to distorted or displaced vertebrae. It can help release trapped nerves and relieve the pain associated with them, as well as ease muscle spasm and help back and neck ache.

In oriental medicine it helps restore proper energy flow in the governing vessel (an extra meridian), which has close connections to the brain and central nervous system.

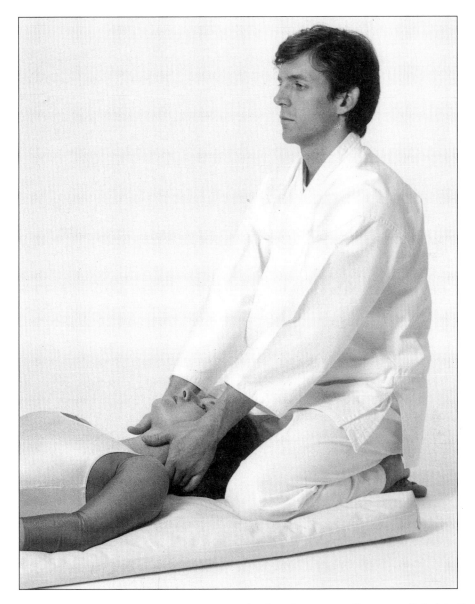

STEP 1 ▲

After finishing work on both your partner's arms, come to kneel above their head, facing their feet. Cup their neck in both hands, allowing the little finger edge of your palm to 'catch' under the ridge of the occipital bone. Now straighten your arms and lean your body weight backwards, applying a gentle stretch which should be felt all the way down the spine. Watch their toes to see if you are stretching the whole body (the toes will move slightly). Repeat the stretch several times. You can also gently massage the back of the neck with your fingers from this position.

Now release the neck and turn it gently to one side, cupping the underside in the palm of one hand and getting ready to give thumb pressure to the upper side with your other hand....

NECK PRESSURE AND STRETCH

In the sitting position you were able to give pressure and stretches to the side and back of the neck. Now that your partner is lying face up, you can reach round to the front of the neck also. Here, however, unlike the sides and back where you were pressing on large, strong muscles, you will be working directly on and beside the cartilage which forms the windpipe. This is very delicate, and your pressure must be correspondingly sensitive. Remember that when your partner's head is turned to one side the windpipe doesn't move with it, and what may seem like the side of the neck is in fact the centre!

Always press very gently at first and get used to the feel of the area. Bone and cartilage naturally feel very different from muscle.

When turning the head to expose the side of the neck for pressure work, give maximum support with both hands on each side. Many people will find it hard just to 'let go' and allow their head to be manipulated freely, so the less hesitant you are the more they will trust you and begin to relax. During the neck stretch many people tense their muscles and try to lift their own head to help you. It is vital that you get them to relax their neck completely before attempting this movement.

THE BENEFITS

I have already mentioned some of the benefits of neck Shiatsu in the sitting position (see page 38). The side and back of the neck sequences shown there are particularly useful in dealing with stiffness, dizziness, headaches, ringing in the ears, insomnia, sore eyes and hangovers. In the sequences shown here, pressure to the front of the neck is effective for influencing blood pressure and relieving heart pains, insomnia, headache and toothache. It also affects thyroid function, and in oriental medicine stimulates the lung and stomach meridians. In general, though, because of the abundance of energy flow in many meridians passing through such a small area, it is easy for 'Ki' to stagnate or become blocked, in turn causing stiffness in the neck muscles and leading to pain.

In addition, the neck is an integral part of the spine and as such is affected by any postural imbalances in other parts of the body. Habit-forming postures such as sitting cross-legged, 'slouching', sticking your bottom out, wearing high-heeled shoes or carrying heavy shoulder bags will often distort the spine in different places and set up a chain reaction which will affect the neck. Shiatsu can help alleviate much of the tension caused by such postural imbalance.

STEP 1 ▶

After finishing the spine stretch, turn your partner's head gently but confidently to one side until they reach their natural stretch point. Cupping the underside of the head in one hand, palm placed over the ear, put the other hand on the side of the neck, fingers firmly supporting round the back, thumb in position just in front of the large muscle which crosses the front of the neck. Now give gentle leaning pressure, distributing your weight equally over thumb and fingers, along the three lines shown on the diagram. Repeat this sequence on the other side of the neck, giving pressure along each line twice.

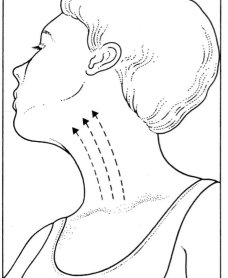

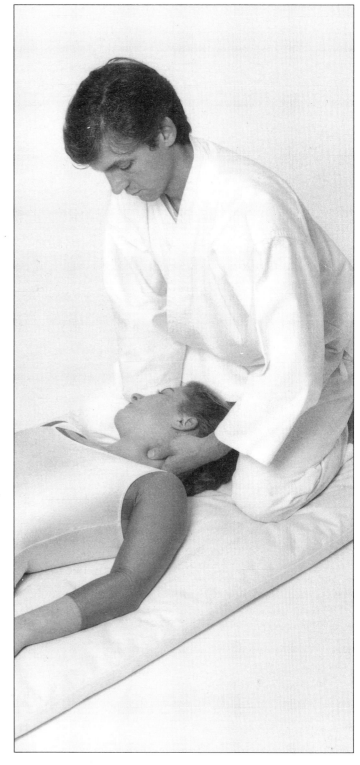

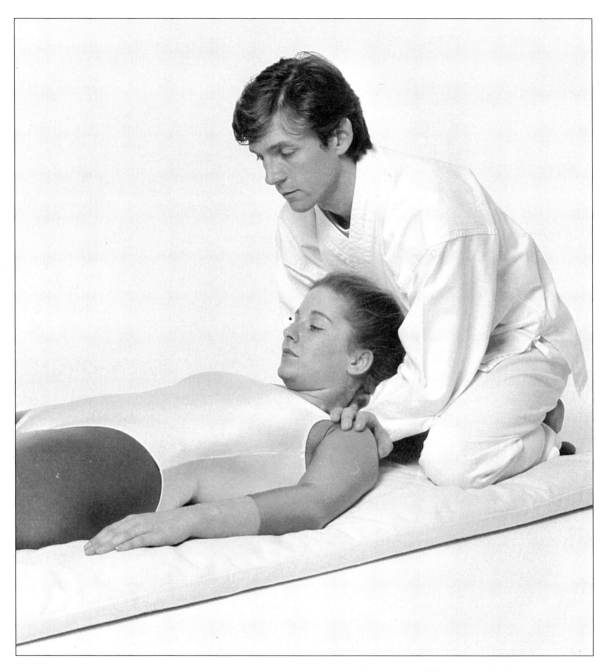

STEP 2 ▲

Return your partner's head to the central position again and gently rock it back and forth in your hands to make sure the neck is loose and relaxed. Lean forward and down and tuck your left forearm under the back of your partner's neck. Bring your left hand up and across to rest on the front of their right shoulder. Now bring your right forearm under your left in the opposite direction so that your arms are crossed, and bring the right hand up to rest on the front of their left shoulder.

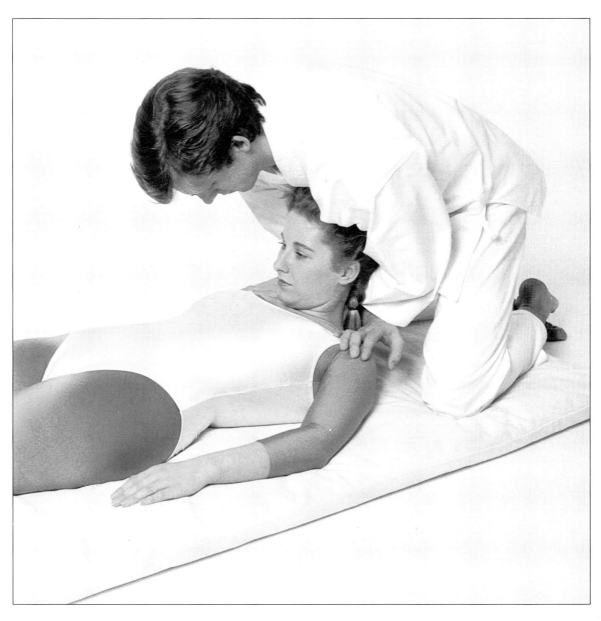

STEP 3 ▲

Making sure that your palm support on the front of your partner's shoulders is firm and that the back of their head is gently but firmly supported in your crossed forearms, kneel up, bringing your body weight up and over towards their feet. This will lift their head and give a stretch to the back of the neck which you can control with the range of your body movement.

Don't overstretch, and make sure the movement is stable and that their chin moves directly towards their chest. If it is more comfortable for you, try the same movement with your arms crossed in the other direction.

After finishing the stretch, replace your partner's head on the floor and get ready to give Shiatsu to the face....

FACE AND HEAD

These sequences can be used as a mini-Shiatsu in themselves and, as with work on the hands and feet, they have a strong effect on the body as a whole. I have put facial Shiatsu towards the end of the book as the face can carry much of the body's overall tension and takes longer to relax than most other muscle groups. So relaxing the rest of the body first will often reduce tension in the face.

Technically, face Shiatsu is a mixture of pressure and massage-like strokes. Since you are working directly on the skin, which is unusual for Shiatsu, it feels good to include some gentle stroking and smoothing over the skin surface. For such a small area you naturally use the thumbs and fingers, still applying your body weight in the same way rather than squeezing with the hands, but taking great care to adjust your pressure according to each area – some, such as the eyes, teeth and ears, are highly sensitive. Because of the natural curves of the face and head, constantly change the positioning of your support hands to allow perpendicular pressure to be applied. Simply follow the sequences shown and apply the usual principles, and you will find these movements effortless and smooth-flowing.

THE BENEFITS

Everyone loves a face massage! There are more muscles in the face than in any other single part of the body. Tension can easily creep into this area, not least because we often put a 'brave face' on things for the benefit of others, creating tension between how we present ourselves to the outside world and how we really are. As such, our face acts as a kind of physical and emotional barometer, reflecting our state of mind and body in spite of ourselves.

Practitioners of oriental medicine have developed a subtle art of diagnosing constitutional and daily health problems from the face, and Shiatsu treatment is said to stimulate normal functioning of the internal organs as well as improve the quality and tone of the skin. Specifically, Shiatsu to the face and head stimulates the urinary bladder, triple heater, gall bladder, stomach, and large and small intestines – all the six Yang meridians of the body – and can help relieve symptoms such as sinusitis, blurred vision, toothache, facial paralysis, headaches and facial tics, as well as improving muscle tone in the face.

STEP 1

After finishing the neck stretch, lay your partner's head back on the floor. Place your palms on either side of their head, lightly pressing them together and tuning into their breathing. Hold this position for a few moments, and allow yourself and your partner to relax completely.

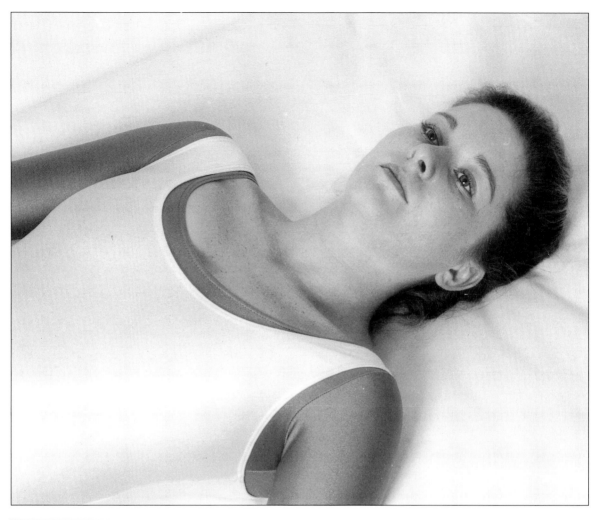

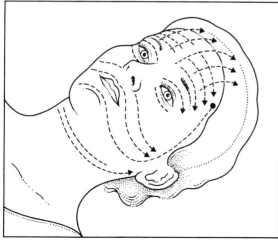

STEP 2 ▶

Now begin to give thumb pressure along all the lines shown in the diagram, starting on the forehead and working down to the chin. Use both thumbs at the same time, and change your finger support to suit the position. For example, finger support is at the sides of your partner's head when giving pressure over the forehead and around the eye sockets. But it is around the side of the jawbones when giving pressure to the upper and lower jaw. Finally, the fingers themselves are used to give pulling pressure under the jaw itself. (See opposite page.)

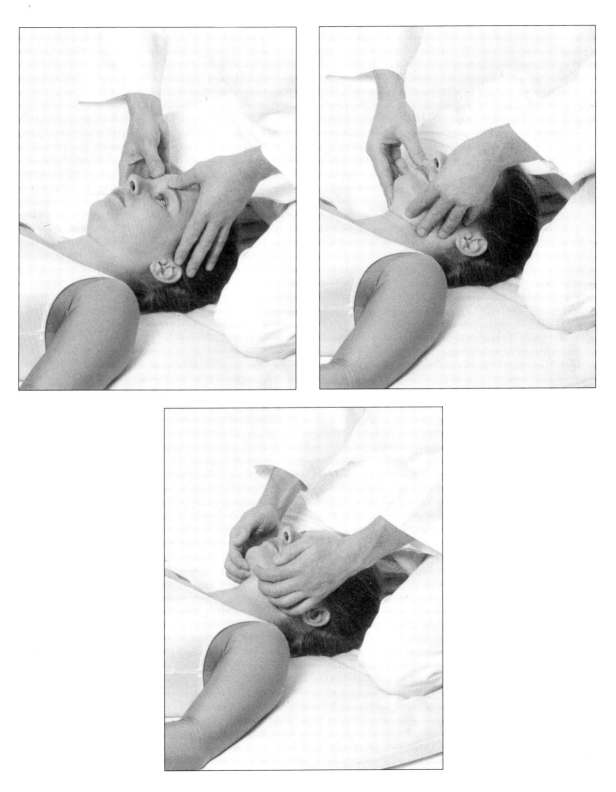

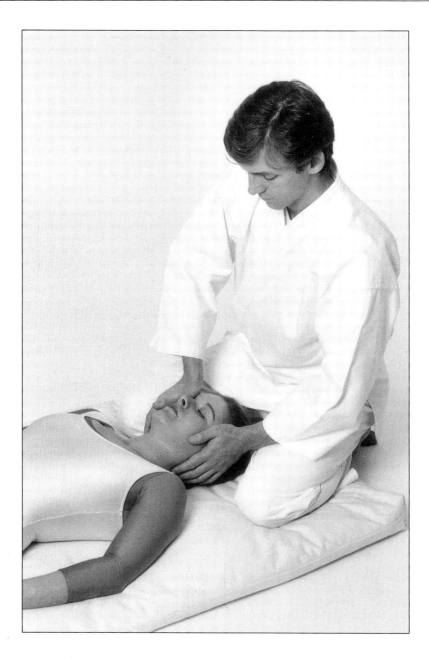

STEP 3 ▲

After finishing pressure along all the lines on the face, support one side of your partner's head with one hand and place the heel of your other hand very gently over one of their (closed) eyes, fitting it into the eye socket. Provided your partner is not wearing contact lenses, a small amount of pressure and gentle rotation of the eyeball is perfectly safe. Repeat the same movement with the other eye.

STEP 4▶

Now take both of your partner's ears between your palm and your fingers and, gently squeezing, lean down so that both ears are stretched. You can do the same to the ear lobes between your thumbs and forefingers.

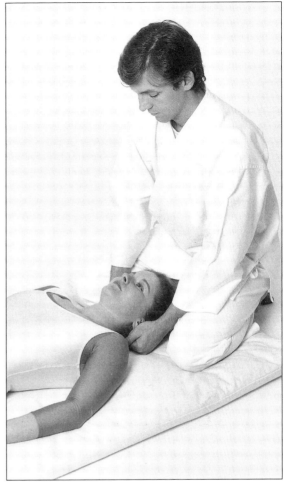

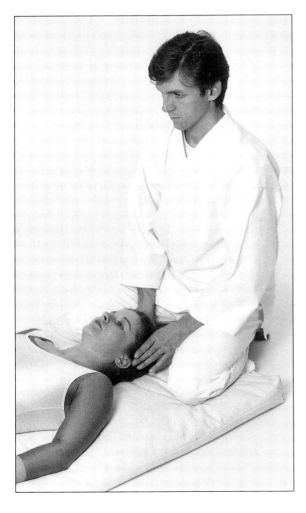

STEP 5◀

Finally, place both hands over the top of your partner's head, fingers wrapped around the sides above the ears and thumbs crossed on a point at the apex of the head on the midline. This point is usually very close to the crown of the head. Lean in and give firm pressure here for a few moments, gradually releasing your thumbs little by little until you 'float off' the head completely.

After releasing the point at the crown of the head lean forward, placing both palms on the front of your partner's shoulders, ready to work on their chest. . . .

CHEST

Like the abdomen, the chest is usually an extremely vulnerable area for most people and work here is best left until the end of your treatment. Pressure should be firm but not oppressive and you should coordinate your movements with your partner's breathing, applying pressure when they breathe out and relaxing as they inhale. Naturally, pressure is given between the ribs and not on them, though it can be applied along the breastbone (sternum) itself (see Step 3 on page 138).

Once again, good finger support is necessary to distribute your weight evenly and to avoid too much pressure being concentrated on your thumbs. When doing chest Shiatsu on a woman, take care to alter the angle of your finger support in order to avoid any direct pressure on the breasts. Take care also when working down the lower part of the ribcage towards the abdomen – it is not so strong in this area, and gentle pressure only should be used.

THE BENEFITS

In oriental medicine the lungs are associated emotionally with communication and expression, the heart with joy, humour and radiance. In people with hunched shoulders and a hollow, sunken chest these functions often seem sad, withheld and lacking in sparkle, as if they are grieving over something or are unable to let their emotions 'out of the bag' – Shiatsu to the chest area can often trigger strong emotional release in people, and you should be aware of this when treating them. Physically, of course, chest Shiatsu benefits the function of the heart and lungs, relieving heart and rib pain, asthma and oppressed breathing; it can also help improve lactation in breast-feeding women.

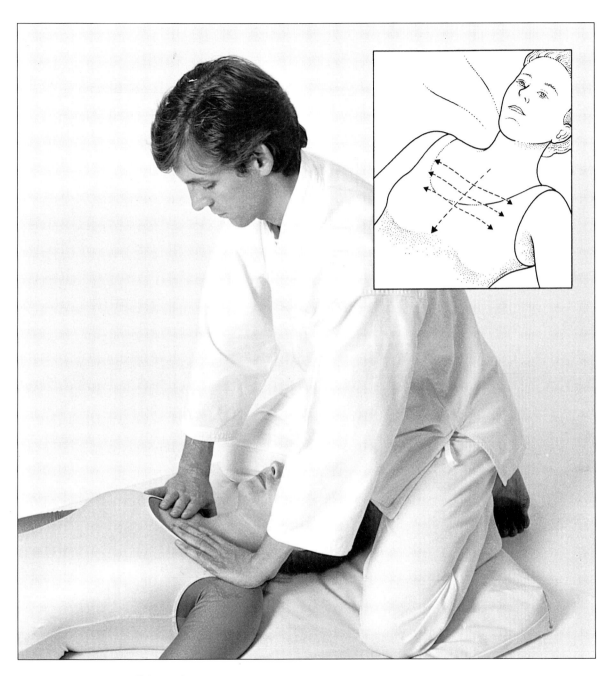

STEP 1 ▲

After releasing the point at the crown of the head, lean forward, placing both palms on your partner's upper chest. With your fingers turned in towards the breastbone, lean forward and apply pressure evenly to the area of the upper chest.

STEP 2▶

Now release your palms and place the thumbs in the first space between the ribs on the upper chest, either side of the breastbone. Using proper support with your fingers, begin to give thumb Shiatsu horizontally along each space between the ribs from the centre of the chest outwards. Follow the lines in the diagram on page 137.

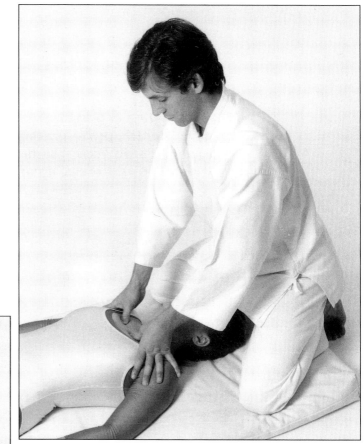

STEP 3◀

Now cross your thumbs one on top of the other and place them at the top of the breastbone. Place your fingers further down towards the abdomen and begin to give thumb pressure down the breastbone from top to bottom, kneeling up as you go so as to maintain perpendicular pressure. Ease your pressure off as you reach the bottom end of the bone, which is quite fragile and sensitive.

After finishing work on the chest, kneel up and place both palms on your partner's shoulders, ready to 'walk' down their arms. . . .

ARM 'WALK', STRETCH AND SHAKE

The palming down the arms here is similar to that done in the prone position (see page 64), and the stretch is similar to the full body stretch done in the sitting position (see page 48).

The palms are facing up for the palm 'walk' and you should take care not to smother your partner as you lean over them with your body. The arm stretch is done using only the weight of your body leaning back, rather like in the leg stretch in the supine position (see page 102). The arm shake should be done with you gently swaying your body first left, then right, and with straight arms, allowing your body movement to lift each of your partner's shoulders off the ground alternately. These sequences should flow one into another and complete the final loosening and opening up of the chest and shoulders before finishing your treatment.

THE BENEFITS

The palm pressure and stretch to the arms works mainly on the three arm Yin meridians, the lung, heart constrictor and heart. These meridians have the function of circulating 'Ki' and blood through the body and all originate in the upper chest, which is powerfully stretched and opened during the sequences. This will improve breathing and circulation and relieve any feelings of oppression in the chest. The arm shake is effective at loosening the shoulders and relieving any residual tension lingering there.

STEP 1 ▶

Having finished work on the chest, kneel up and place both palms on the front of your partner's shoulders. Now begin 'walking' down towards the hands, giving pressure to the insides of their arms as far as the palms. Lean your body weight forward as you go.

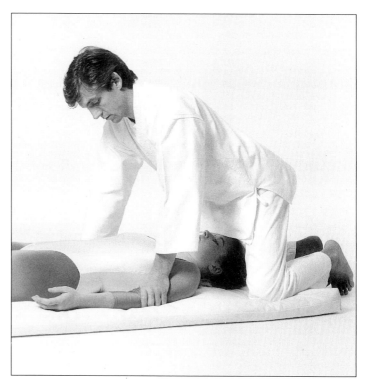

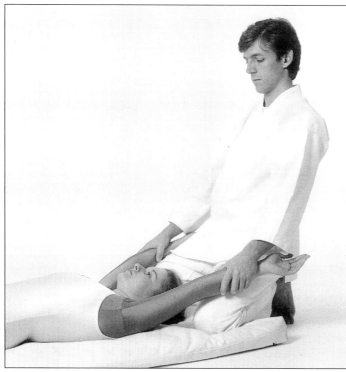

STEP 2 ◀

When you reach the palms, take hold of your partner's wrists and sit back on to your heels, bringing their arms over their head to rest on your thighs. From here, either lean straight back to give the stretch or, rolling back on to your toes, bring your knees up and lean back, resting their forearms on your knees. In either case, your partner should feel an arm as well as a chest opening stretch. (See also the photograph at top of page 141.)

STEP 3 ▶ ▼

Use your partner's 'dead weight' to counterbalance you as you lean back and up, coming up into the standing position in a smooth, arc-like movement. Place your feet either side of your partner's head so that you are standing directly above them.

In the process of standing up, slide your hands from their wrists to their palms so that you end up palm to palm. Now begin to sway your body weight from side to side, keeping your arms straight, and gently lift your partner's shoulders off the ground alternately. You can vary the speed of this movement to give a good shake to the arms and shoulders.

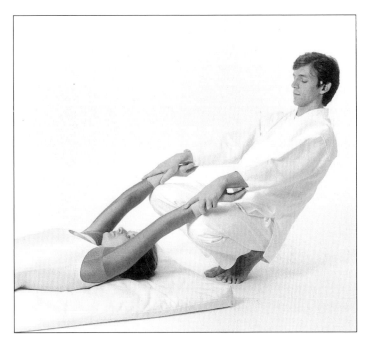

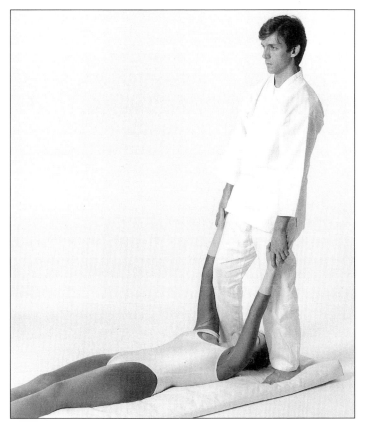

Now return your partner's left hand to the floor, walk around to their right side, still holding the right hand, and come to kneel alongside them, one hand on the Hara....

HARA

The significance of the abdomen or 'Hara' in Japanese was discussed at the beginning of the supine position (see page 92 and also page 30). In medical practice it is used as part of the diagnostic process as well as in treatment. However, since it is one of the most vulnerable areas of our bodies we are often very protective of it. At the end of a treatment, when your partner has had plenty of time to relax their whole body, is often the most likely moment for work in this area to be well received. I have included only the very simplest of sequences in this book as Shiatsu in this area demands quite a lot of skill and practice.

You should not give Hara Shiatsu if your partner has just eaten (in fact, Shiatsu should not be given at all on a full stomach) or if menstruating (though very gentle pressure is all right).

Your pressure must be particularly smooth and gentle when working here – avoid any sudden, sharp movements. Even just the warmth and comfort of the palm placed on the abdomen for some time can be very calming and invigorating at the same time. Tune into your partner's breathing and apply pressure when they breathe out, releasing again as they breathe in.

THE BENEFITS

The benefits of Hara Shiatsu are widespread since all meridians pass through here and the major organs of the body are all located here; thus it is the vital centre of our physical and emotional being. Stimulating this area directly will affect all the body systems. In particular, though, it will help with disorders such as cramps, poor digestion, loss of appetite, indigestion and constipation. It is also good for regulating menstruation and stopping menstrual pains and cramps. It can regulate urination and help with kidney problems.

Finally, the Hara is the centre of one's energetic being. Shiatsu here will help balance and restore overall energy levels, especially sexual energy, desire and potency.

STEP 1 ▶

Having come round to sit at your partner's right side after finishing the arm shakes, place your right palm gently on their abdomen, quietly tuning into their breathing rhythm. After a few moments, begin gently pressing the fingers of your hand over different areas of the abdomen, noticing if any of them feel particularly soft or weak. In these areas, place your thumbs one on top of the other and, supporting with your fingers on both sides, lean your body weight gently in and begin to give pressure to these points. With each one, find the maximum depth of pressure, hold for a few seconds and then very gradually begin releasing your thumbs each time your partner breathes in, finally allowing your hands to 'float' off your partner's body before moving to the next point.

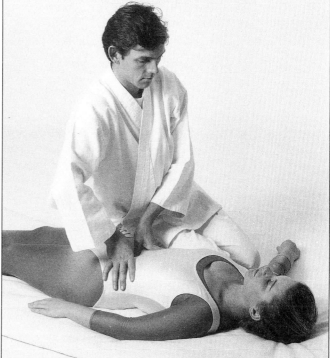

STEP 2 ◀

Having finished giving pressure to the points you have chosen, place your right palm on your partner's abdomen once more and rest it there for some time. When you are ready to take it off, release it in the same way as the thumbs each time your partner breathes in, until your palm gradually lifts off the body.

Now cover your partner with a blanket and let them rest for fifteen minutes or so. Do not leave them alone in the room if they fall asleep, as they may be disorientated when they wake and you should be there to reassure them. Advise them it is best not to indulge in any major activity for two hours or so after the treatment – this includes hot baths. You may mention that they should sleep well and will feel very relaxed and that this will usually be followed by a feeling of renewed vigour.

Ask them back again!

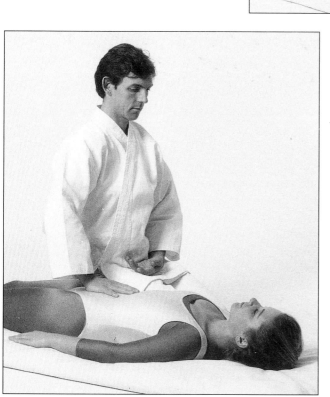

BIBLIOGRAPHY

Capra, Fritjof *The Tao of Physics* (Berkley: Shambala)

Dawes, Nigel and Harrold, Fiona *Massage Cures* (Thorsons)

von Durkheim, Karlfreid *Hara – the Vital Centre of Man* (Unwin Paperbacks)

Kinoshita, Haruto *Illustration of Acupoints* (Ido No Nippon Sha)

Masunaga, Shizuto *Zen Imagery Exercises* (Japan Publications)

Masunaga, Shizuto *Zen Shiatsu* (Japan Publications)

Moore, Charles A., Ed. *The Japanese Mind* (University of Hawaii Press)

Ohashi, Wataru *Do It Yourself Shiatsu* (Unwin Paperbacks)

Roshi, Yamada *Introductory Lectures on Zen Practice* (San Un Zendo, Kamakura)

Sergel, David *Macrobiotic Way of Zen Shiatsu* (Japan Publications)

Various *Essentials of Chinese Acupuncture* (Foreign Language Press, Beijing)

Veith, Ilza *The Yellow Emperor's Classic of Internal Medicine* (University of California Press)

USEFUL ADDRESSES

To obtain further information on the style of Shiatsu illustrated in this book, including a full-length video cassette demonstrating all the sequences, as well as classes and treatments, contact:

The London College of Shiatsu
Dugdale House
Santers Lane
Potters Bar
Herts EN6 2BZ
UK
Tel: 0707 647351
Fax: 0707 646613

Or: Nigel Dawes
162 E. 90 Apt. 5R
New York
NY 10128
USA
Tel: (212) 369 3247
Fax: (212) 410 0927

To get a copy of the Shiatsu Society handbook which lists all registered practitioners of Shiatsu in Britain, or to find out more information on the schools in Britain and abroad as well as to apply for membership and receive the quarterly Shiatsu newsletter, contact:

The Shiatsu Society
5 Foxcote
Wokingham
Berks RG11 3PG
UK

Tel: 0734 730836